in_focus

Fixing
Health
Systems

2nd Edition

in_focus

IDRC's *in_focus* Collection tackles current and pressing issues in international development. Each publication distills IDRC's research experience with an eye to drawing out important lessons, observations, and recommendations. Each also serves as a focal point for an IDRC website that probes more deeply into the issue, and is constructed to serve the differing information needs of IDRC's various readers. A full list of *in_focus* websites may be found at **www.idrc.ca/in_focus**. Each *in_focus* book may be browsed and ordered online at **www.idrc.ca/books**.

IDRC welcomes any feedback on this publication. Please direct your comments to The Publisher at **info@idrc.ca**.

in_**focus**

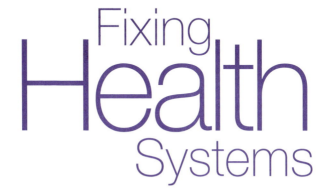

Fixing
Health
Systems

2nd Edition

by **Don de Savigny, Harun Kasale,
Conrad Mbuya,** and **Graham Reid**

INTERNATIONAL DEVELOPMENT RESEARCH CENTRE
Ottawa • Cairo • Dakar • Montevideo • Nairobi • New Delhi • Singapore

In collaboration with the Ministry of Health and Social Work, Tanzania

Published by the International Development Research Centre
PO Box 8500, Ottawa, ON, Canada K1G 3H9
www.idrc.ca

© International Development Research Centre 2008
First edition 2004

Library and Archives Canada Cataloguing in Publication

Fixing health systems / by Don de Savigny ... [et al.]. – 2nd ed.

"In collaboration with the Ministry of Health, Tanzania".
Available also on the Internet.
Issued also in French under title: La réforme du système de santé.
Includes bibliographical references.
ISBN 978-1-55250-409-3

1. Tanzania Essential Health Intervention Project. 2. Medical policy —
Tanzania. 3. Rural health — Tanzania. 4. Health planning — Tanzania.
5. Public health administration — Tanzania. 6. Health planning —
Developing countries. I. De Savigny, Don II. International Development
Research Centre (Canada) III. Tanzania. Wizara ya Afya

RA395.T34H42 2008   362.1'0425709678   C2008-980090-7
ISBN (e-book) 978-1-55250-411-6

IDRC Books endeavours to produce environmentally friendly publications.
All paper used is recycled or comes from responsibly managed forests, and
is recyclable. All inks and coatings are vegetable-based products.

This book is an integral part of IDRC's thematic website on the Tanzania
Essential Health Interventions Project: **www.idrc.ca/in_focus_tehip**.
The full text of the book is available online and leads the reader into a
virtual web of resources that explores the TEHIP story.

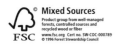

Mixed Sources
Product group from well-managed
forests, controlled sources and
recycled wood or fiber
www.fsc.org Cert no. SW-COC-000789
© 1996 Forest Stewardship Council
FSC

Contents

In Africa, health care has been in a state of crisis for several decades. The Tanzania Essential Health Interventions Project (TEHIP) has sought to test a premise that called for health reforms based not just on increased funding but on more strategic investments in health.

Two large districts in Tanzania — already engaged in health reforms centred on devolving management of resources to the local level — attempt to bring health spending more in line with cost-effective approaches to the local disease burden. Information from Demographic Surveillance Systems makes it possible for planners to determine spending priorities. A series of simple management tools enable those district planners to allot funds to interventions that will have a greater impact on local causes of mortality.

Chapter 3. The Results ➤ **45**

New means of planning lead district health teams to budget more proportionally to address major contributors to mortality such as malaria and a cluster of childhood illnesses. Effectively addressing those problems, however, requires that a modest funding top-up be applied to increasing capacity within the health system. This allows for better training, more effective deployment of resources such as drugs, better clinical practice, and increased patient satisfaction. The overall result is a dramatic decline in mortality in the two districts.

Chapter 4. Extending TEHIP's Innovation and Impact ➤ **71**

The two districts' success in substantially lowering mortality demands that the tools for achieving that success be disseminated more widely, both within Tanzania and internationally. This section of the book documents current efforts to extend the impact of the TEHIP innovations.

Chapter 5. Lessons Learned ➤ **77**

The primary lesson arising from the TEHIP experience is that investing in health systems is an effective way of improving population health. This chapter presents the critical lessons learned from the TEHIP experience.

Epilogue. TEHIP Maintains its Momentum ➤ **85**

As TEHIP approached the end of its 8-year lifespan, the TEHIP team came to realize that the most difficult work was, in a sense, just beginning.

Foreword

On the web
THE ISSUE

The challenges that face Africa in the sphere of health care are formidable and often daunting. After decades of stagnant or worsening poverty and health indicators across the continent, the Millennium Development Goals (MDGs) — adopted by the United Nations at its Millennium Summit of September 2000 — have set benchmarks for improvements in the health picture. If accomplished, the MDGs would represent major advances in the well-being and survival rate of millions of people. Those goals envision that by 2015 child mortality can be reduced by two thirds, that maternal mortality can be reduced by three quarters, and that infectious diseases such as malaria, tuberculosis, and HIV/AIDS — which threaten to do even more damage tomorrow than they do today — can be held in check and indeed reversed.

Are these goals realistic? In Tanzania, recent experience in the large rural districts of Rufiji and Morogoro gives us cause for optimism. Over 4 years, child mortality within these districts (with a combined population of more than 700 000) has fallen by more than 40%, which puts them well on the way to achieving the MDG related to child health. We attribute these gains not to a single intervention but to a range of simple measures to improve health system efficiency and to allocate health funds more in proportion to the local causes of mortality (quantified using data collected from Demographic Surveillance Systems).

The underlying proposition behind this achievement — that health could be significantly improved by adopting a minimum package of health interventions to respond directly, and cost-effectively, to evidence about the local burden of disease — was one of the key proposals put forward in the *World Development Report 1993: Investing in Health* (World Bank 1993). Around the same time, Tanzania was embarking on health reforms centering on the decentralization of health planning authority (which would enable districts to allocate funds more in line with local health needs). Therefore, it made sense for Tanzania to accept an offer to host the Essential Health Interventions Project, which aimed to test the *World Development Report 1993*'s central hypothesis.

In the beginning, no one could have made an intelligent guess at what the outcome of that initiative would be. Today, however, we can clearly state that we have been overwhelmed by the results of that decision. Using a series of interrelated management tools created by the Tanzania Essential Health Interventions Project, or TEHIP (as the project would become known), district health teams have been able to vastly improve their local health systems' efficiency, leading to startling health improvements such as the dramatic reduction in child mortality mentioned above. Those tools — of which there are more than originally envisioned — continue to be indispensable to the districts' health planning. They allow district health planners to do much more with the marginal increases in funding currently available — proving that it is possible to begin to improve health significantly while working for more substantial increases in budgets, provided that resources are allocated more rationally and the **system** is strengthened.

In the coming years, the enhanced performance of the overall health system may prove to be a critical cornerstone for new initiatives in health care, as countries such as Tanzania adopt new therapies and treatments for HIV/AIDS, for instance. It is obvious that good management, motivated health workers, and functional networks of communication and transportation are required for such new treatments to reach the people who need them and for those treatments to be used effectively.

On the web
THE ISSUE

Given the dramatic successes achieved in the Rufiji and Morogoro districts, it is a moral imperative for Tanzania and its health partners to support the widespread promotion and dissemination of the very tools and strategies that led to those improvements and to address the immediate and recurring problem of "going to national scale" with the toolkit. We have already made a start on this by expanding to an additional 9 districts, which together constitute the two entire regions of Coast and Morogoro. However, there is an urgent need to facilitate practical and cost-effective national scaling up by improving the pre-service and in-service training "machinery."

As this book goes to press, the Ministry of Health is moving ahead, within its TEHIP partnership, to provide a plan and a budget for a consolidated and strengthened Ministry of Health Zonal Training Centre Network around the country. In the immediate term, however, it will be crucial to keep the momentum going as we move from "best practice" to national scale-up. It is vital that these dramatic improvements in district health systems not only reach all corners of this large country of Tanzania but also our neighbours in the countries that constitute sub-Saharan Africa and, for that matter, all the nations of the world. For, as we all know, diseases recognize no borders and successes in any one country should be shared.

It is my sincere hope that this book will promote and strengthen the case that evidence-based planning and prioritization, combined with simple tools to improve health system delivery, is a strategy that makes sense. It is a strategy that challenges communities to forge robust partnerships for the future and it holds great promise for other developing countries confronting similar challenges.

M.J. Mwaffisi (Ms)
Permanent Secretary, Ministry of Health,
United Republic of Tanzania

August 2004

Preface to the
Second Edition

In November 2008, a Ministerial Forum on Research for Health in Bamako, Mali will take stock of the strides that have been made since the first Ministerial Summit on Health Research was held in Mexico City in 2004. That gathering focused the world's attention on the importance of strengthening health systems and implementing health policy that is informed by reliable research. It is fitting that the first edition of *Fixing Health Systems* was launched at the Mexico City Summit, since the book details ongoing efforts in Tanzania to achieve those very things: local health systems efficient enough to deliver treatment to the people who need it, and evidence-based health policy that directs resources toward the most critical challenges.

The 4 years since that Summit have seen this focus on health systems move from being a novel, even marginal idea, to something that now approaches the status of conventional wisdom. This change in outlook is reflected in the multitude of new efforts to improve the mechanics of health care delivery.

New initiatives have been introduced that aim to revitalize health systems by improving training and support for health workers. The need for sound data as the basis for policy is being addressed by groups such as the Health Metrics Network and the Alliance for Health Policy and Systems Research, both of which are now firmly ensconced within the World Health Organization (WHO). Both established and new donors are supporting research and capacity strengthening for health systems and, increasingly, bilateral donors are recognizing that operational research must be integrated into core health systems support. Indeed, as this publication goes to press, IDRC and the Alliance for Health Policy and Systems Research are preparing for the Bamako forum by examining how closely current funding allocations match the intent to support health system research and the strengthening of health systems, and what gaps should be addressed. Meanwhile, an increasing number of initiatives around the world are grappling with the challenges of real-time, rigorous evaluation and, where possible, pragmatic randomized controlled trials of health systems and social interventions.

In Africa, it is — paradoxically — the moral imperative to provide treatment for a single disease that has brought into sharp relief the crucial need to strengthen all aspects of health systems. HIV/AIDS highlights the necessity of having a range of functional services and capabilities in place. One of the more obvious and widely publicized of these is the provision of affordable and widely accessible drugs. But dealing with HIV/AIDS also requires the training, deployment, supervision, and adequate compensation of health workers; laboratory facilities to diagnose disease and track viral resistance; supply chains that can bring medicines to wherever they are needed; access to unstigmatizing facilities; programs to promote prevention and proper nutrition for patients; and, of course, respectful palliative care. Without such a functioning, full-spectrum system, essential services and treatments will remain out of reach, and patients in need will go untreated.

The exact same challenges have been encountered by the major multilateral initiatives set up to address epidemic levels of tuberculosis and malaria. It is ironic that increasing verticalization of health interventions has finally led almost full circle to the vision of comprehensive primary health care, which captured the world's imagination at Alma-Ata in 1978. The forthcoming report of the WHO Commission on the Social Determinants of Health will once again cast a spotlight on a much broader range of health determinants and health interventions. It is tempting to think that the international health community is finally moving beyond the quest for simple silver-bullet solutions to complex and changing problems.

On the web
THE ISSUE

But how is such a comprehensive vision and approach to be realized? The Tanzanian Essential Health Interventions Project (TEHIP) was and remains a compelling and practical example. This book, describing how TEHIP played out on the ground, remains as relevant today as it was when it was first published. This second edition, therefore, contains, unchanged, the full original text, together with its foreword, preface, recommendations, and appendices.

But in the 4 years since the publication of *Fixing Health Systems*, new lessons have emerged about how to institutionalize change. The post-TEHIP experience demonstrates how the new ideas and practices emerging from a robust and ambitious project can be integrated into the everyday dynamics, politics, and processes of a national health system. This second edition, therefore, includes not only this new Preface but also an Epilogue, which tells the story of what happened next, and how and why it happened. It also points to new lessons about managing the transition from pilot project to everyday practice.

The Epilogue also raises new questions and new challenges facing those of us who are committed to improving health and increasing health equity. Central among these is a new level of a long-standing challenge: how to analyze and address the often "taboo" issues of both big "P" and little "p" politics. Taking initiatives up to scale brings different actors together and requires negotiation across different skill sets and sectors. Ultimately, it is important that all participants in this process — those with roles both mundane and exotic — understand their contribution to the broader project and remain motivated to play their part.

Finally, the Epilogue raises a more sobering new challenge. The dark shadow attached to the realization of how much a project like TEHIP can do in reducing rates of death and disease (in this case, primarily among under-5s), is the revelation of how much more remains to be done. There is still too much readily treatable and preventable illness that has not yet been addressed. Yet the message here is one of confidence and determination. The "low hanging fruit" — that is, the most obvious areas where mortality and morbidity can be reduced — is pretty well gone (in the Tanzanian case, at least). Now it's time to build some new ladders and start picking the fruit that's harder to reach.

TEHIP and the TEHIP story provide excellent ideas and tools for this challenge.

Christina Zarowsky
International Development Research Centre
February 2008

Preface to the First Edition

The phrase that best describes the attitude emerging from the decade-long experience of the Tanzania Essential Health Interventions Project (TEHIP) is "cautious optimism."

The hopefulness stems mostly from the fact that TEHIP has produced good news about a subject where the outlook invariably has been bleak. The essential aim of the project — which evolved as a unique collaboration between Tanzania's Ministry of Health and Canada's International Development Research Centre (IDRC) — was to test a proposition put forth in the World Bank's *World Development Report 1993*. That report suggested that mortality and morbidity rates in developing countries could be significantly reduced even with modest resources if health care funding was allocated to cost-effective health interventions more in line with the prevailing local "burden of disease."

More than 10 years on, the TEHIP experience indicates that this idea is indeed solid. In two Tanzanian districts, annual budgets are recast to address the local burden of disease — targeting funds on a more selective list of health interventions in proportion to the impact of specific diseases. The resulting improvements in the health picture in those districts have dramatic, encouraging implications. They confirm that many deaths that currently occur in developing countries are preventable. They show that we have the knowledge to deliver better quality health care (and thereby to save lives) now, without waiting for additional expenditure or the design of new drugs and vaccines.

In the course of arriving at these conclusions, the project has also developed a set of practical managerial and technical tools that can be adapted to fit other health care settings and potentially be put into use in other developing countries. TEHIP provides model approaches that can be adapted for use in a variety of circumstances — and which cannot be dismissed as a one-time anomaly.

Meanwhile, the "caution" in that phrase "cautious optimism" stems from a number of factors, not least of which is the realization that "scaling up" the project's innovations (as requested by the Ministry of Health) remains a daunting task. In addition, we are well aware that some of the lessons learned over the course of the project's work appear to contradict current conventional wisdom. For example, our direct involvement with district health managers has convinced us of the necessity of taking an "integrated" approach to health care reform — that is, to combine new interventions into coherent packages that make practical, everyday sense to health care practitioners at the village level and upwards. However, much of the world seems to be moving in the opposite direction: opting for a "vertical"' approach that seeks to improve health by dealing with diseases individually, in isolation, one at a time. This, we believe, frequently results in a fragmentation of service delivery that puts extra stress on the all-important health system and especially the health care worker on the front line. Such weakened delivery of essential health care compromises the ability of the health system to reduce the burden of disease.

Invariably, this subject of reform and support to health systems in Africa comes down not to abstract theoretical formulations but to real people in real situations. Consider, for example, the tables and charts that appear throughout this book, documenting changing mortality rates in two Tanzanian test districts, Rufiji and Morogoro. As you look at those graphics, we urge you not to think about the pictures you see as numbers or statistics. Instead, think about them as representations of real people — people with families that grieve, people who had rich lives before them, people who should have lived.

For years, development workers have encouraged people who once would have been silent to contribute their ideas and perspectives — they seek out the "community voice" and the voices of the disenfranchised. You can think of those thick black lines on paper as an important contribution by people who died too soon because of inadequate health care. The experiences of the dead should be heeded as much as those of the living. That many of those people died from illnesses that could have been cured or prevented — if the health system had adequate resources and capacity — is tragic. Yet, it is hoped that we will find some solace if learning from their fate — understanding why they died and how the health system failed them — helps prevent similar needless deaths in the future. We need to discern the patterns behind those deaths, so that others can live longer and healthier lives.

TEHIP expresses its profound gratitude to the people and health care providers of Morogoro and Rufiji districts, who accomplished

On the web
THE ISSUE

so much and who made the achievements documented in this book possible. Full details of individual acknowledgements are included in Appendix 1.

Don de Savigny
Research Manager, Tanzania Essential Health Interventions Project
International Development Research Centre, Canada

Harun Kasale
Project Coordinator, Tanzania Essential Health Interventions Project
Ministry of Health, Tanzania

Conrad Mbuya
Research Coordinator, Tanzania Essential Health Interventions Project
Ministry of Health, Tanzania

Graham Reid
Project Manager, Tanzania Essential Health Interventions Project
International Development Research Centre, Canada

August 2004

Don de Savigny is now Head of the Health Systems Interventions Research Unit at the Swiss Tropical Institute.

Harun Kasale and **Conrad Mbuya** are, respectively, Lead Consultant and Consultant for the National Expansion of TEHIP Tools and the Strengthening of Zonal Health Resource Centres, Ministry of Health and Social Work, Tanzania.

Graham Reid is now Senior Program Specialist at IDRC's office in Nairobi.

Chapter 1

The Idea

On the web
THE ISSUE

For several decades now, Tanzania — like most other countries in sub-Saharan Africa — has faced the dual burden of a crisis in public health and a grave shortage of resources with which to address this escalating, interlocking web of problems.

The health challenges confronting most of Africa have been well publicized: high on the list are the spread of deadly diseases and problems such as malaria, HIV/AIDS, tuberculosis, malnutrition, and anemia. Almost equally well known is that the effects of these devastating epidemics are exacerbated by conditions of poverty. Poor citizens are caught, in effect, in a vicious cycle: while their poverty makes them more vulnerable to the effects of illness and less able to afford proper treatment, succumbing to sickness in turn reduces their already-meager capacity to generate income.

Both aspects of this cycle can be seen as factors in the national context in Tanzania. While it has struggled with the onslaught of infectious diseases, high rates of child mortality, and widespread disability, Tanzania (one of the poorest countries in the world, with an annual per capita income of US $280) has until recently only been able to allot roughly US $6–8 per person annually to health care (Table 1). By comparison, according to Conference Board of Canada (2004) figures, Canada spends an annual US $2 809 per capita on health care, while annual per capita health care expenditures in the United States total US $4 819.

The experience of the Tanzania Essential Health Interventions Project (TEHIP) suggests, however, that sudden injections of funding alone will not necessarily solve the health care crises facing the nations of Africa — although certainly funding for health systems and health interventions must increase substantially over time. Nor is a panacea likely to be found in new and more effective drugs and vaccines — although these innovations are also an important component in the battle to improve health for populations in the developing world. Instead, the project's experience makes clear that a critical missing link in reducing high levels of morbidity and mortality in developing countries is a system-level intervention: the ability to allocate health resources in strategic ways that target real and prevailing needs, and that enable health planners and individual health workers to operate more effectively at the level of the front line health facility. In other words, the efficiency of the health system (and the appropriateness of strategies in health care) is key to translating health care spending into an increase in health gains.

The policy implication we draw from this is that institutions and agencies concerned with improving the currently grim health outlook in Africa must take a more systemic approach — turning at least some of their attention to apparently mundane matters within the health system, such as infrastructure,

> Institutions and agencies concerned with improving the currently grim health outlook in Africa must take a more systemic approach.

Table 1. A profile of selected health-relevant indicators for Tanzania (circa 2002)

Indicator	Statistic[a]	Source
Population	34.4 million	Tanzanian census, 2002[b]
Urban–rural population ratio	34:66	UN Population Division[c]
Gross national income	US $280 per capita	World Bank[c]
Health spending	US $11.37 per capita	Tanzania Ministry of Finance (2001)
Inflation	19% per year	World Bank[c]
Adult literacy	84% of males 67% of females	UNESCO[c]
Total fertility	5.2 children per woman	UN Population Division[c]
Infant mortality	104 per 1 000 live births	UNICEF (2004)
Child <5 mortality	165 per 1 000 live births	UNICEF (2004)
Maternal mortality	5.3 per 1 000 live births	Tanzania Ministry of Health (2002)
Life expectancy at birth	44 years	UN Population Division[c]
Low birth weight	13% < 2 500 g	Tanzania Bureau of Statistics and Macro International (1999)
Child <5 underweight	29% (moderate and severe)	Tanzania Bureau of Statistics and Macro International (1999)
Child labour	32% of 5–15 year olds	Tanzania Bureau of Statistics and Macro International (1999)
Primary school enrollment	47% of required age group	UNESCO[c]
Poverty head count	36% below US $1 per day	Tanzania (2003)
Inequity ratios of poorest to least poor quintiles for		
- Health outcomes (mortality)	Av. 1.7 x worse in poorest	Gwatkin et al. (2000)
- Health interventions (access)	Av. 1.6 x less in poorest	Gwatkin et al. (2000)
Population per health facility	7 431	Tanzania Ministry of Health (2002)

(continued)

Table 1. concluded

Indicator	Statistic[a]	Source
Ill or injured in previous 4 weeks	28.3% of population	Tanzania Bureau of Statistics (2003)
Health service utilization	69% of illness or injury episodes	Tanzania Bureau of Statistics (2003)
Access to health facilities	93% live within 1 hour	Tanzania Ministry of Health (2002)
Access to improved drinking water	68% of population	Tanzania Bureau of Statistics and Macro International (1999)
Access to oral rehydration	21% of children with diarrhoea	Tanzania Bureau of Statistics and Macro International (1999)
Access to immunization (measles)	89% of children by age 1 year	UNICEF (2004)
Access to vitamin A supplements	93% of children 6–59 months	UNICEF (2004)
Access to antenatal care	49% of pregnancies	Tanzania Bureau of Statistics and Macro International (1999)
Access to antimalarial drugs	53% of children with fever	Tanzania Bureau of Statistics and Macro International (1999)
Malaria deaths	>100 000 per year	Tanzania Ministry of Health (2002)
HIV/AIDS prevalence	7.6% of 15–49 year olds	UNAIDS[c]
Health and civil service reforms	Underway	Tanzania Ministry of Health (2002)
Sector-wide approach (SWAp) to financing	Underway	Tanzania Ministry of Health (2002)
Decentralized health basket funding	Underway	Tanzania Ministry of Health (2002)

[a] All statistics are from 2002 or represent the most recent estimate.
[b] See http://www.tanzania.go.tz/census/.
[c] As quoted in UNICEF (2004).

training, capacity building, human resources, and health planning, that form the foundation for future advances in the well-being of Africa's citizens.

A history of hope and struggle

The story that unfolds in the pages ahead holds lessons that we believe can be applied widely throughout the developing world. At the same time, however, this is a narrative largely rooted within the specific geographical setting of Tanzania, a land of spectacular contrasts that range from the mountain forests of Kilimanjaro to arid plains, coastal deltas, and sun-soaked beaches. Indeed, these contrasts become immediately apparent by comparing the two districts within which TEHIP's work unfolded. Whereas Morogoro district is mountainous and lush, Rufiji is characterized both by a mostly dry, flat expanse in its interior and by a tidal delta on its coastline.

As enchanting as this landscape is, it has also served as the backdrop for a tragic and all too familiar story. Like their counterparts in countries across Africa, Tanzanians have suffered through a grave health crisis for the better part of a generation. While the full force of new or resurgent infectious diseases — most notably malaria, HIV/AIDS, and tuberculosis — has brutally rearranged the social landscape of an entire continent, national health systems have been wholly unable to meet this challenge, sometimes teetering on the brink of collapse.

In the specific case of Tanzania, it is especially and bitterly ironic that this health care crisis has occurred despite longstanding policies that had placed health care high on the national agenda. Since its launch as an independent unified country in 1964 (the product of an amalgamation of two former British protectorates, Zanzibar and Tanganyika), Tanzania, under the first postindependence government of Julius Nyerere, sought to ensure that Tanzania's citizens had access to education, health care, and clean water. Plans to provide these amenities and services centered on a new and unique social contract, whereby citizens who relocated to modern villages (typically taking the form of a collection of small hamlets) became the beneficiaries of government programs. Each village had pumped water, a school, and access to a clinic — most often these facilities were built by volunteer labour from within those communities. The government kept up its end of the bargain by agreeing to maintain those structures and by dispatching teachers to the schools and health workers, drugs, and supplies to the new health facilities. This agreement led to new health care machinery being set in motion: medical training centres were built and large numbers of graduates poured out into the rural areas to provide the health care that the government had declared a public right.

While this momentum continued through the 1970s and into the 1980s, by the mid-80s the system was foundering. Arguably, part of the problem was that centrally planned health care management had been inefficient and unresponsive and was unable to maintain the health care infrastructure (such as the village dispensaries).

Yet another and indisputably massive factor in the erosion of Tanzania's health system was the international debt crisis that in the 1980s was creating similar disruption throughout the developing world. Economies dependant upon the export of natural resources were crippled by the twin scourges of dramatically falling commodity prices and rising interest rates that caused the debts of developing nations to increase exponentially virtually overnight. At the height of the debt crisis, Tanzania, like other developing countries, was faced with onerous — perhaps impossible — debt-repayment demands while its export income plummeted. With close to half of government revenues being channeled toward debt repayment — at the expense of domestic social spending — the negative impacts on Tanzania's health care system were dramatic and prolonged. Funds for training health staff and maintaining facilities were no longer available. Many clinics had no drugs or health supplies on the shelves. Wages were eroded by inflation, devaluation of the local currency, and by continuing austerity measures. Many health workers continued to perform their duties without receiving a salary. There were cases where facilities were operated by unqualified staff after the local clinician had died or simply left.

Early attempts to revive the system were unsuccessful. The introduction of user fees and other cost-recovery measures — intended to infuse new funds into the system — only served to drive more Tanzanians out of the orbit of the health care delivery system. People who had been unhappy with the low quality of services provided now became indignant at being asked to pay for those same low-quality services. Similarly, support from the international community began to wane as the outlook for health care in Africa became bleaker and "donor fatigue" began to set in.

On the web
THE ISSUE

Bold new initiatives

In Tanzania, as elsewhere in Africa, there is more hope today than existed during the darkest days of the mid-1980s to the early 1990s. Emblematic of the new ideas and new optimism that has been injected into the debate over health care in Africa is the 2001 report of the Commission on Macroeconomics and Health, which was formed by the World Health Organization (WHO) in 2000 to examine the relationships between health, development, and social equity, and to recommend measures to minimize poverty and maximize economic development. The world has also seen significant new funding and institutional muscle being applied to the problem of infectious disease, as exemplified by the Global Fund to Fight AIDS, Tuberculosis and Malaria. This major new funder was established in January 2002 as the outgrowth of work undertaken by the G-8 group of countries, leaders of African states, and UN Secretary General Kofi Annan. In addition, institutions such as the Bill and Melinda Gates Foundation, the Rockefeller Foundation, the United Nations Foundation, and the Roll Back Malaria Partnership have made health care in Africa a high priority at a time when international development programs have also redoubled their efforts on the continent. These are all positive and highly desirable initiatives reflecting a new political will to help deal with Africa's health reform challenges and representing international recognition of the need to commit the appropriate resources to that goal.

At the same time, however, echoes of the old era of structural adjustment programs — designed to impose fiscal austerity on developing countries during the debt crisis — continue to exert a restraining influence on national health care systems. For example, externally mandated hiring freezes still make it difficult for many countries to recruit new health practitioners necessary to staff their health facilities. Wages of health workers in many developing countries remain desperately inadequate, to the point where critically important public servants in many countries must consider other forms of work or working abroad to earn a living wage. The era of structural adjustment may be over, but the effects of earlier damage continue to cast a long shadow.

This presents a striking and disturbing paradox: at a time when major new funds are being promised for new therapies, technologies, and health interventions, the prospect is that those same funds will be channeled through weakened, fragile national health systems that remain inefficient, inadequate, and under-funded. A lack of ground-level capacity may well hamper the grand designs conceived of at the international level. Consider the potential obstacles, for instance, involved with bringing antiretroviral drugs to Africa to treat HIV/AIDS. Getting those drugs onto the dispensary shelves and into the hands of people who need them will

> At a time when major new funds are being promised, the prospect is that those same funds will be funneled through weakened, fragile national health systems.

require health systems that have information, communication, transportation, diagnostic, and human resource capacities sufficient to move the drugs to the right places, in the right numbers, at the right times, to the right people, and with the right counseling and follow-up.

TEHIP's piece of the puzzle

A central preoccupation of TEHIP has been to learn how a functioning and efficient health care system — one with resources logically targeted at the most pressing health needs of the population — could contribute to significant improvements in the health of the population. Essentially, the project's goals have been to help local authorities fix the gross technical and allocative inefficiencies that characterized health care delivery in two rural Tanzanian districts and, related to that, to help bring proportional spending into line with actual needs. The project has facilitated this process by encouraging an "evidence-based" approach — that is, by promoting the use of evidence about the local-level burden of disease (as measured through mortality) and evidence on cost-effectiveness as the main determinants of how to establish priorities in health care budgeting.

This idea — that increasing the overall effectiveness of public health services could have a major impact on the overall health of the population — is not new. Before the effects of structural adjustment took hold in the 1980s, several influential reports emphasized the need for a focus on primary health care and strengthening of comprehensive health systems to reach the people in need and to improve health outcomes. Those documents included the 1978 *Declaration of Alma-Ata* (WHO and UNICEF 1978) and UNICEF's Child Survival Revolution initiative of 1982 (see UNICEF 1996) — both of which stressed the need for equity, participation, and a multisectoral systemic approach to improving health.

After many years of crisis in the 1980s, a variation on that basic perspective re-entered the public eye with the publication of the World Bank's 1993 edition of its *World Development Report* (WDR93). In what appeared to be a reversal of previous Bank policy stressing fiscal restraint and drastic cuts to public sector programs, WDR93 proposed that increasing investments in health was key to economic development. It also prescribed that such investments should be based on evidence that would target and focus cost-effective interventions on the local "burden of disease" that exists in a particular ecosystem. For example, in an area where malaria accounts for 40% of the burden of disease, allocating only 5% of the budget would be inadequate for treatment and prevention. There is a natural tendency in human nature to put 80% of our efforts on 20% of the problem. In health systems, this leads to huge inefficiencies and low impacts.

Using this general principle of bringing efforts more in line with the weight of the problems, WDR93 proposed specific minimum packages of essential and primary health care interventions. The World Bank speculated that by taking this targeted "evidence-based" approach (wherein the burden of disease and cost-effectiveness become the determining factors of how budgets are spent, rather than administrative or political considerations or simple guess-work), relatively small funding increases could produce significant and tangible improvements, simply through correcting prevailing technical and allocative inefficiencies. Calculations included in WDR93 suggested that raising per capita public spending on health in low-income countries to US $12 annually — a modest sum, but still higher than existing funding levels in Tanzania and neighbouring countries — should lead to a 25% decline in the burden of disease. In short, WDR93 argued that, although increasing health funding is critical, the method by which those funds are allocated is also crucial to ensuring that new funding produces substantial improvements in health outcomes (Bobadilla et al. 1994).

Although the logic of WDR93 was generally well received, the report sparked very little discussion as to how this promising theoretical premise could be translated into practice. Notably absent from the report were answers to any of the "how" questions. How could local authorities get a true picture of the existing burden of disease? How could the new information be used to reengineer local health systems — in other words, what mechanisms could be devised to allow decentralized planners to incorporate burden of disease into their work in a manageable and practical way? Essentially, TEHIP was created to answer the "how" questions. Conceived in October 1993, its aim has been to develop and test a set of simple, user-friendly tools to enable local-level health planners to plan on the basis of evidence.

The experiment has now run its course: the planning tools that evolved from several years of collaboration between local authorities and TEHIP have been put into use in two Tanzanian districts with populations totaling 741 000 — a sample large enough to make it difficult to dismiss the results in these districts as the outcome of an "experiment" that would be difficult to replicate in "real life." Since 1997, District Health Management Teams (DHMTs) in the rural districts of Morogoro and Rufiji have been using an expanding tool kit to plan and implement health services to more precisely respond to local evidence. Concurrently, DHMTs have been assisted in their attempts to revamp their health systems by the provision of a financial top-up that brought their health budgets closer to WDR93's annual US $12 per capita target.

The results of these changes have been dramatic, with the two districts having witnessed marked improvement in health outcomes in the wake of the introduction of new planning methods and modest budget top-ups in the order of an additional US $1 per capita. In Rufiji and Morogoro, for example, child mortality fell by over

In Rufiji and Morogoro, child mortality fell by over 40% in the 5 years following the introduction of evidence-based planning.

40% in the 5 years following the introduction of evidence-based planning (Figure 1). In the same period, the death rate for Rufiji adolescents and adults between 15 and 60 years old declined by 18%. Corresponding figures for districts that have not been using the planning tools — and indeed all across most of Africa — have been stagnant, at best, for children and increasing for adults. From neighbouring comparison districts, cross-references have been made with other contextual factors (such as differences in levels of rainfall, disease outbreaks, and health risks) that are known to affect mortality rates. Those factors do not appear responsible for the declining death rates in this case.

The results from the two planning districts, therefore, support the earlier predictions in WDR93. Health system adjustments correlating health spending with burden of disease and cost-effectiveness do allow for significant improvement in health with modest increases in expenditures. Furthermore, we have no reason to believe that this result should be considered unique to the particular rural Tanzanian setting. The planning tools used by district health planners and managers are fully adaptable and can be used — given the appropriate local statistical inputs — by district health planners in other country settings.

Testing a potent idea

The process that ultimately led to the development and deployment of TEHIP's health planning tools began in October 1993, when Canada's International Development Research Centre (IDRC) convened an international conference in Aylmer, Quebec, Canada. Representatives of the World Bank, WHO, UNICEF, and other multilateral and bilateral organizations, nongovernmental organizations, universities, and ministries of health were asked to consider whether it would be possible to test the idea that evidence-based health planning could produce efficiencies that would lead to positive improvements in local health. They answered in the affirmative.

Child <5 mortality
per 1 000 live births

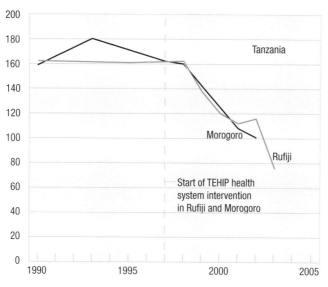

Figure 1. Reversing the trend in child mortality after district-level health system interventions in Tanzania. Sources: National Sentinel Surveillance System, Ministry of Health Tanzania; Coastal Sentinel Demographic Surveillance System (TEHIP Rufiji DSS for 1999 to 2003); Central-East Sentinel Demographic Surveillance System (AMMP Morogoro DSS for 1992 to 2003); Tanzania Demographic and Health Survey 1992 for 1990 local baselines in Morogoro and Rufiji; Tanzania Demographic and Health Survey 1996 for 1995 baseline in Rufiji; UNICEF for Tanzania national under-five mortality trend (http://www.childinfo.org/cmr/revis/db2.htm).

Subsequently, IDRC and the Canadian International Development Agency (CIDA) provided funding to launch what was then known as the Essential Health Interventions Project, or EHIP, (the lack of a "T" denoting that Tanzania had not yet been identified as the host country, and the Tanzanian Ministry of Health had not yet become a partner in the enterprise). The following 3 years saw a series of international meetings intended to collect as wide an array of expert input as possible and to refine the research design. The first meeting of EHIP's advisory committee, hosted by WHO, took place in Geneva in January 1994. There were 9 subsequent meetings in various cities culminating in the drafting of a "scope"' document in March 1996 (see TEHIP 1998), a call for proposals, and the final approval of research proposals in December of the same year.

This process of discussing and defining the parameters of research was much more exhaustive than is the norm — most development initiatives would have much stricter timelines attached and less latitude to deal with theoretical concerns. However, there was a general feeling that since the program aimed to test an idea and approach that were potentially groundbreaking, and likely contentious, it was imperative to take time to "get it right" by exploring all the potential implications and pitfalls from the outset and by thoroughly thinking through the design model. This development and design phase of the project relied on high-level international and domestic expertise. When fieldwork began in Tanzania, however, direction came almost exclusively from local authorities and most funding went into the modest annual per capita incremental health budgets for the 741 000 residents of the two districts. The daunting challenge facing these small groups of district managers is underscored by that population figure. Expressed another way, 741 000 is a population greater than that of 66 (close to one third) of the world's countries (the population of Guyana, for example, is 705 000). Furthermore, this large population is spread over an area almost the size of Switzerland, with varied and often difficult terrain. Given the scope of their challenge, it is clear to us that the accomplishments of the district teams could indeed hold lessons for entire countries.

> The accomplishments of the district teams could indeed hold lessons for entire countries.

Understanding how this work led to actual changes in health care delivery in Rufiji and Morogoro requires recounting the particular stages in the project's life cycle. The first phase, noted above, was one of broad-based consultation that took place between 1993 and 1996. In 1994, the Tanzanian Ministry of Health responded positively to an invitation to participate — triggering the selection of Tanzania as the research site, the engagement of the Ministry as a partner in the project, and the reorientation of EHIP to TEHIP. From this point, discussion began on how the research program could be made compatible with the specific circumstances of health care delivery in Tanzania.

Tanzania was interested in participating in the program largely because it had embarked on a program of health reforms receptive to decentralized, evidence-based planning and wanted to know how it could be implemented. A cornerstone of the Tanzanian health ministry's plans to reform the health system was the devolution to local authorities of health care delivery and management responsibilities, accomplished through the creation of District Health Management Teams (DHMTs) (see box: "More responsive planning through DHMTs"). TEHIP — with its emphasis on decentralized control over health budgets — would provide an opportunity to test whether the strategy being considered by the Tanzanian Ministry of Health was sound.

When the design phase concluded in December 1996, a second phase emerged, which involved setting up Demographic Surveillance Systems (DSSs) to collect comprehensive data on mortality to calculate the prevailing burden of disease in Rufiji and Morogoro. Although originally intended to monitor the impact of evidence-based planning, this data soon became part of the raw material TEHIP would use to create the "tool kit" intended for use by health managers.

Another aspect of the work involved putting the finished tools — as they became available — into the hands of the DHMTs. Once the project was designed and the tool kit progressively assembled, TEHIP scrupulously avoided interfering in how district health authorities used those tools or spent their money. Furthermore, additional funds flowing to Rufiji and Morogoro only consisted of top-up funds amounting to approximately US $1 per capita annually, which was needed to bring the districts closer to the minimum spending levels suggested in WDR93. (DHMTs could spend the additional funds not only on strategic interventions but also partly on initiatives that would make the health system more functional — for instance, by upgrading management and administrative skills, increasing internal transport and communications capacity, or repairing substandard facilities). The only other advantage DHMTs enjoyed — besides the additional funds — was increasing access to the developing tool kit.

Complexity anchored by fundamental questions

TEHIP evolved into a uniquely multifaceted and complex program integrating both research and development functions, employing the skills of Tanzanian researchers and practitioners, and examining a wide array of specific health care questions. During the course of this evolution, however, project workers would always come back to a series of questions and principles that defined the scope of the work and pointed toward its goals and potential outcomes.

One of the major results of those early years of research design and thorough consultation was the formulation of three interrelated questions that would serve to keep the project on course as its work proceeded:

➤ How and to what extent can decentralized district health plans be more evidence-based?

➤ How and to what extent can evidence-based plans be implemented by decentralized health systems?

➤ How, to what extent, and at what cost can such evidence-based plans have an impact on population health?

It is significant that, given the repeated use of the phrase "how and to what extent," these questions contain within them qualified rather than definitive statements. This reflects the project's assumption that health systems could never be managed **entirely** on the basis of evidence — political factors, subjective judgments, and windfall opportunities will always intrude. Still, the intent was to ensure that evidence — detailing the true burden of disease at the local level — becomes as powerful a factor as possible in the allocation of health care resources. The aim was to move away from the norm of health care policy formation in developing countries, where spending is often dictated by numerous secondary factors that have little to do with the prevalence of disease or with a logical plan for maximizing health. Prominent among these factors is bureaucratic inertia — the pressure to simply replicate the proportional allotments of last year's budget, added to or subtracted from the current year's financial picture. The paradigm advanced by donor agencies is another persuasive factor. Few health officials find it easy to turn down external funding aimed at, for example, a specific disease — even if that particular disease is not a significant concern in the area and addressing it could divert attention and resources from more pressing population needs.

In addition to this key principle that evidence should guide health policy and resource allocation, there were other operational principles that emerged during the first consultative phase of the project. One such principle was that resources should be controlled by local authorities rather than by a central office. Another was that district management teams should be able to allocate those resources. These principles were reinforced by circumstances within Tanzania and by emerging policy trends in the field of international development. For instance, as we've already noted, Tanzania had committed itself to decentralization as part of its package of health care reforms. Donor agencies were also changing their approach: many had abandoned the practice of stipulating that funds should be spent in specific ways. The new practice — adopted by some national development agencies — of providing funding to be allotted by the recipient governments according to their reading of the most pressing need is known as the "sector-wide approach" (SWAp). The project's practice of providing DHMTs with a basket of funds — which the teams would then divide to respond to the picture that emerged from the evidence — was very much a precursor of the SWAp strategy for decentralized district health basket funding.

The need for an integrated approach

TEHIP was also guided by another principle that — although it was not spelled out initially in the formal design of the project — became clearer as time elapsed and as field experience accumulated. As the project's base of operations moved to Tanzania, it became increasingly obvious that any set of prescriptions for reforming health care delivery would have to keep the community-level health worker foremost in mind. The reality at the village level is that a dispensary or health centre will have one or perhaps two workers responsible for the care of thousands of people and for every aspect of the facility's operation. These one or two people shoulder a tremendous responsibility — the success or failure of programs designed elsewhere comes down to how well those individual health workers can incorporate those imported plans into their daily routine. It therefore became obvious that any new initiatives should be seen as part of a complete package that makes organizational sense for the overburdened health worker. The more complicated and taxing the individual remedy becomes, the less likely that those remedies will succeed.

In response to this reality, our approach was to look for what we would call "integrated" solutions to problems. The integrated approach took many forms. It influenced methods of treating patients by suggesting that health care should address the overall condition of the patient and should not be directed in isolation toward diagnosing and dealing with specific individual diseases. It influenced the reorientation of health systems by stressing innovations and initiatives that could be integrated into the routines of community health workers and managers. It also had a major influence over how TEHIP as an organization was structured.

> Health care should address the overall condition of the patient and should not be directed in isolation toward diagnosing and dealing with specific individual diseases.

In the next chapter, which describes the development and deployment of the tools, we will see numerous examples of this integration-oriented approach at work. For example, a guiding idea was that diagnostic tools should be kept simple. TEHIP was aware that it would be impractical for busy managers and health workers to use tools that presented too much information or burdened them with unnecessary complexity. The tools steered district priorities toward health interventions that formed "bundles" or "packages" — which had the potential to deal more efficiently with overlapping or coexisting health problems — as opposed to "stand alone" health interventions that dealt with single diseases on an individual basis. The rationale was that complementary and integrated sets of treatments would be easier for front-line workers to use and, therefore, were more likely to be successful.

This integrated approach contrasts with what is often termed the "vertical" model. We use this term to describe what we see as top-down efforts to control particular diseases, one at a time. Such programs often involve directives from high levels of authority, issued without adequate consideration for how the community-level health worker can integrate these new activities and responsibilities or how new initiatives will fit in with the prevailing local burden of disease or the structure and capacities of the local health system. We see the vertical approaches and campaigns as gaining momentum in an era when large amounts of money are flowing into international disease-control programs. This new funding creates tremendous pressure to be able to demonstrate results quickly and thereby creates a bias against taking a longer term, more systemic approach to health care.

Indeed, the integrated approach seems to run contrary to several established patterns that exert a powerful influence over the formation of health policy. In academia and within bureaucracies, there are few incentives to take an integrated approach that keeps the needs of the peripheral, front-line health worker and local manager in mind.

This bias against an integrated approach has a clear impact in the field. For example, the typical way of training health workers has been to take them out of the clinical setting to provide them with a few days of training on one particular disease, on an individual basis. TEHIP has taken the contrary stance, believing that it is better to train workers systemically — training them to look at a range of signs and symptoms as indicators of a number of possible conditions. This approach makes particular sense in an environment where patients often suffer from more than one illness and where common symptoms may point to the presence of more than one disease.

Another example of the integrated mentality at work is internal: the connection between the project's "research" and "development" functions. Research to establish the burden of disease in the districts, to gauge the ways in which health budgets are allocated, and to determine how best the public can interact with the health system was undertaken simultaneously with the development and deployment of the tools. Both aspects of the program were meant to be complementary and mutually reinforcing. This is very different from the standard model in which research and development remain distinct entities with different staffing, separate budgets, and little communication between the two. Normally, after research has suggested a particular policy direction, additional funds must be raised to construct a pilot project and thereby translate the new ideas into actual change. Since TEHIP was a well-funded "research and development"' project operating within the context of a functioning, living health system, it could roll those normally separate functions into one package: providing DHMTs with access to relevant research and then enabling them to act upon those findings annually in subsequent planning cycles. Research was undertaken, tools for the DHMT managers were developed, and the tools were used to change the way the health system was managed and health care delivered at the community level — all of this occurring within the same project cycle. In fact, the cycle continued after the tools had been put into practice. Ongoing research allowed for the creation of a kind of "feedback loop" that enabled practitioners to examine whether the tools and systemic changes were working, to refine and modify their developments, and to consider the development of new tools at any stage as the need for them became apparent.

Efficiency leads to equity

A final philosophical note to add, before we examine specific contributions, is that the project's work must be seen in the context of the sometimes-competing concepts of "efficiency" and "equity." The project's emphasis on efficiency — its focus on maximizing the cost-effectiveness of health care spending — should not be viewed as some cold-hearted accounting exercise. Rather, it was a means to an end, adopted specifically as a way of making the system more equitable.

There are two ways of assisting the poor through public spending. One way is to concentrate on the "distributional" issues — for example, by creating programs that target "the poorest of the poor." Another means is to focus on the "production" issues — in this case, that meant retooling the health system so it became capable of producing higher levels of health across all segments of society.

In other words, the reforms aimed to buttress the "universal" nature of this social benefit. Taking this approach made eminent sense in a situation — such as existed in Rufiji and Morogoro — where an inefficient health system produced consistently poor results and where most people were uniformly poor. Now, all citizens can go to the local clinic with a reasonable expectation of getting appropriate treatment for the most important population health problems. In reality, though, the biggest impact of increasing the efficiency of these universal health services is on the poor. This is because, in a country where the majority of people are poor, a minimum package of essential interventions addressing the diseases that account for the largest segments of the burden of disease will by definition benefit the poor. It is the poor who suffer the most from these diseases (such as malaria), so it is the poor who have the most to gain. Conversely, since the diseases that disproportionately affect the rich (such as cancer) did not appear as significant in burden of disease statistics, those diseases did not absorb significant resources within those intervention packages. Therefore, one effective consequence of such an approach is a transfer of public health care resources from the rich, who can afford private health care, to the poor, who rely exclusively on the public system.

Still, there is a small minority of rural poor that has not been positively affected by health care changes in Rufiji and Morogoro. Now that it has been demonstrated that "health production" issues can be effectively addressed, policymakers in Tanzania may well want to return to unfinished business and consider adopting a much more deliberate focus on equity — that is, to pay "the equity premium" to widen the distribution of health care to those who still have not benefited from the ongoing health reforms. Our use of that phrase "the equity premium" acknowledges the reality that reaching the most marginal or remote subset of the population will not likely be accomplished in a "cost-effective" manner. Reaching this difficult-to-reach subset (let's assume it comprises 10% of the population) may cost as much as extending effective health services from 30% to 80% of the population. The extra cost does not change the fact, however, that achieving greater equity in the distribution of health care benefits is a desirable social goal that may be worth the additional expense. Pursuit of such a goal will be more effective when added to a system that has corrected its gross inefficiencies.

Chapter 2

The Approach

When TEHIP began its operations in Tanzania, its management team set up shop in a large room in the newly renovated offices of Tanzania's National Institute of Medical Research in Dar es Salaam. This made TEHIP a neighbour of the Ministry of Health, the Tanzanian offices of the World Health Organization, and the Tanzania Public Health Association — appropriate circumstances for a project that sought to influence the formation of health policy at both the national and international levels. This cluster of offices — a nerve centre for the health sector in Tanzania — is a short distance away from the shoreline where the turquoise waters of the Indian Ocean meet the city of Dar es Salaam.

More noteworthy than the natural setting, however, was the scene inside the project's office. In contrast to the established norms in Tanzania (and in many other countries around the world), TEHIP opted not for individual offices but for an "open concept" plan. This was much more a reflection of management philosophy than an indication of a particular taste in interior design. With no internal walls and no doors (just chest-high partitions separating desks), the physical form of the office made it easier for a multiplicity of contributors to work together, shoulder-to-shoulder, toward a common goal, using diverse but complementary means. This open concept design, in short, facilitated the practice of "comanagement." Within that fluid office space, Tanzanians and international staff, financial and administrative workers, big-picture planners and "details people," researchers and development workers could trade ideas and enlist each other's expertise and support. Meetings did not have to be scheduled — conferences would spontaneously occur as managers turned to face (and raise questions with) their coworkers. This constant exchange of information kept managers "in the loop" about the project in general and about what was happening outside their immediate area of expertise. The open office space also made it impossible for individual agendas to undermine common goals; impossible that "factions" should emerge and compete against each other for influence or dominance.

TEHIP also hoped that its management style — as embodied by the architectural innovations at its project office — would provide an example of what should happen at the district and community levels. The unique organization of the office demonstrated to other contributors within the health system that the formation of cohesive, functional teams could lead to better results, as a wide range of viewpoints and specialties were brought to bear on individual problems. The management team also tried to show through its organizational preferences that minimal resources could be deployed in a way that produces results cost-effectively. For example, the managers who shared a common office space also shared a vehicle. As well, having a program of proper maintenance of office equipment — rather than simply replacing computers, for example — delivered a strong message that the right systemic support could help extend the life and impact of precious investments.

In short, far from being a typical development project, TEHIP sought to be a uniquely collaborative joint venture. In many specific respects, its *modus operandi* was that combining different skills, talents, and perspectives could provide greater strength to the overall enterprise, leading to better results. In the pages that follow, we examine two critical ways in which a diverse range of participants were brought together within new and innovative frameworks.

Integrating research and development

By integrating its research and development aspects into a cohesive, functional whole, the project sought to strengthen and increase the effectiveness of both of those individual facets of the program. The development side — which assigned funds to, and encouraged the implementation of, interventions designed to make district health systems more effective — was strong because its decisions were based on current research, including continuous feedback on how well innovations were working and how they might be improved. Meanwhile, the research side had an immediate policy impact and enjoyed a higher than normal level of credibility within communities because researchers were directly involved in a tangible effort to improve health in the districts. Therefore, researchers were seen not as pursuing an abstract agenda, but as direct contributors to better health.

This practical orientation of TEHIP's research component was exemplified by its use of a "plausibility design." This is distinct from the classical scientific model that painstakingly sets up experiments that control for confounding to prove definitively a relationship between a specific cause and a specific effect. Functioning within a living, dynamic health system — where the process of change was already underway, and where a multitude

On the web
THE RESEARCH

THE APPROACH | **27**

of uncontrollable real-life influences could affect health indicators — TEHIP would never be able to ascribe any positive changes in health outcomes exclusively to the policy changes and interventions it championed. However, by retrospectively comparing health outcomes in the districts with those in neighbouring districts — and by assessing what role other factors such as rainfall disparities, localized disasters, and resource inequality may have played in changes in those outcomes — researchers were able to test the "plausibility" that specific policies contributed to the greatly improved health pictures in Rufiji and Morogoro.

> "A butterfly cannot fly with one wing. Likewise, development cannot be achieved without research."
>
> — Dr Peter Kilima

Dr Peter Kilima, former Director of Preventive Health Services at the Ministry of Health, uses an evocative metaphor to describe the integration of research and development. "A butterfly cannot fly with one wing," he says. "Likewise, development cannot be achieved without research."

How did the "two wings of the butterfly" assist one another? First, the research wing identified major health issues and budgeting priorities. It also provided the foundation for the development of new management tools designed to help the DHMTs base their planning more upon evidence. Then, the development wing applied specific expertise to the development of new information tools and strategic interventions, and provided the budget so that district teams could implement these innovations. Following this, the research wing helped to identify any weaknesses in the tools and new strategies, thereby assisting in their refinement. The development wing adjusted its work to accommodate the new information, and so on. In this way, the butterfly — with its mutually reinforcing and mutually dependent wings — moved forward more quickly and effectively than might otherwise have been the case.

There are indications that this approach of integrating research and development has led to positive changes in the districts. For example, in the post-TEHIP era, the DHMTs have commissioned their own research. This suggests that rather than viewing research either as a threat or as an unhelpful distraction from important daily work, the district teams now acknowledge that research can inform their development initiatives in ways that lead to better results and improved health outcomes.

> District teams now acknowledge that research can inform their development initiatives in ways that lead to better results and improved health outcomes.

The consortium approach

Enlisting the expertise of the best local researchers — skilled in a wide range of specialties — was also a key characteristic of the project's approach. In keeping with IDRC's philosophy, it was always understood that Tanzanians, who were familiar with the country and the realities of working there, would conduct the research. In addition, this collaborative approach suggested that those researchers should be organized cross-institutionally as "consortia." The formation of those consortia began following the call for proposals, when researchers representing the full range of academic institutions in Tanzania were invited to a briefing at a hotel in Dar es Salaam. The assembled researchers organized themselves into several consortia, with each one subsequently being granted small amounts of funding to prepare proposals addressing various health care issues.

During the peer review process that followed, TEHIP's international scientific advisory committee judged the completed submissions according to the applicants' tactical approach to answering the questions — did they suggest innovative, cost-effective ways to tackle the research problems? The committee then selected two successful consortia that included researchers drawn from various institutes in the University of Dar es Salaam, the Muhimbili University College of Health Sciences, and the Ifakara Health Research and Development Centre.

Beyond the advantage to the project of being able to recruit the best people, the consortium approach offered several benefits for the Tanzanian research community. For one, it was most Tanzanian researchers first experience of working inter-institutionally and programatically, where individuals had control over a particular piece of a larger program's research agenda and depended on colleagues in other centres for part of their data. This approach — with people assembled from different departments and different institutions — helps develop trust, professional rapport, and an ability to bring different perspectives to bear on a common problem. It also provides good experience with the "centres of excellence" style of research support that has become common for broader, large-budget research programs in the developed world in recent years.

The research begins

The Tanzanian research consortia moved into the field armed with three core questions (as we observed in Chapter 1) that focused their efforts upon the practicability of taking a more evidence-based approach to health care planning.

- ➤ How and to what extent can Tanzanian district health plans be more evidence-based?

- ➤ How and to what extent can evidence-based plans be implemented by decentralized district systems?

- ➤ How, to what extent, and at what cost can such evidence-based plans have an impact on population health?

At the level of everyday practice, however, there was the need for more specific inquiry about how Tanzania's districts planned, how communities related to the health system, what mortality rate existed in the districts, and what could be done to reduce levels of mortality. To address the need for this information, work was divided into three thematic areas, each supported by a consortium of researchers:

-➤ Health systems — how the district health planning process worked;

-➤ Health behaviours — how the population sought health services; and

-➤ Health impacts — what happened to patients as a result of ill health.

Proceeding simultaneously, the research areas (described below) fed into a broader understanding of how evidence on mortality could lead to more effective health system planning in the districts. Research in these areas also continued during and after the introduction of innovations into the health system. Following the development of the planning tools, the deployment and use of those tools by DHMTs, and the introduction of other innovations within the health system, the research consortia would ask to what extent these innovations were achieving their goals and how they could be modified or improved. With the district health systems in a continual state of transformation, it was the researchers' job to assess the impact of changes on the development side and to continually ask "where do we go from here?"

Research on health systems planning processes

A health systems research consortium was contracted to conduct both quantitative and qualitative studies of the systems and services operating in Rufiji and Morogoro districts and document changes over time. The essential objective of this research was to determine how DHMTs could use locally generated information on mortality, cost-effectiveness, health system capacity, and community preferences in their planning and distribution of health resources. The consortium began by observing and describing which district officials were responsible for planning and how they went about that task. Later, as the project offered DHMTs a series of planning tools to help them plan more on the basis of evidence, the research consortium shifted its focus to examine what impact those tools actually had on planning. Did the availability of the tools lead DHMTs to alter their funding priorities, or did it remain business as usual? Did the tools dispel previous biases in health care planning? Were the tools easy to use? How could the tools be modified to become more effective? What new tools might be developed to deal with unaddressed concerns and unmet needs?

Research on household health-seeking behaviours

This consortium — with team members drawn from a wide range of health disciplines such as anthropology, demography, sociology, systems analysis, economics, and epidemiology — examined a range of issues related to the extent and ways in which citizens used the district health systems. This area of research was based on the idea that even the most dramatic improvements to the health care system would not lead to better population health if clients stayed away from health facilities. The team sought to answer a number of questions. How frequently do people go to health facilities? What makes them decide to go to a facility and what keeps them away? Is there a preference for traditional or modern health care? What do clients think about the quality of care at their local health facility? As innovations were developed and put into use — such as the Integrated Management Cascade (see Chapter 3), designed to increase efficiency and boost local facilities' access to drugs, lab tests, etc. — researchers sought to determine whether levels of use and satisfaction increased.

> Even the most dramatic improvements to the health care system would not lead to better population health if clients stayed away from health facilities.

Some research into when and why clients go to a health facility produced startling results. For example, it had been known that although most people are likely to seek modern care for most forms of fever and malaria, they also generally associate late-stage, life-threatening malarial fever with convulsions — known as *ndegedege* — with evil spirits and changes in weather rather than with malaria. Therefore, at the point at which malaria is most deadly, many Tanzanians were believed to seek out traditional healers rather than modern care. The research showed that this understanding was exaggerated and that most patients did seek modern care as their first resort. The problem now becomes one of making sure this care is of high quality and obtained quickly, rather than wasting efforts on changing beliefs about traditional care.

Research on health impacts

The objective of this research component was to quantify changes in the burden of disease, as measured by mortality, in the two districts under study. Central to the research was the use of Demographic Surveillance Systems (DSSs), which had been set up to gather vital data and track the health of large segments of the populations of Rufiji and Morogoro. Evidence generated by the DSS (which is described below) allowed district officials, firstly, to identify the major contributors to mortality that should be addressed proportionally in the health budgeting process. At the latter stages, the continuing flow of evidence allowed DHMTs to gauge what impact health reforms had on population health.

The Demographic Surveillance System

The "evidence engine" powering health reforms

Functioning as the "evidence engine" that provides the raw materials — the raw data — for the tools, the DSS is a system that has come to play a key role in health planning, not just in Tanzania but increasingly throughout the developing world. In countries where no vital registration system exists, the DSS can serve as a highly reliable mechanism to supply data on burden of disease, mortality, population, household size, and many other key topics. A DSS is rooted in a sentinel area where the entire population is monitored for changes in health status. But the impact of DSS activity is felt much more widely, with information from these sentinel areas used to create representative profiles for other districts. Urban and rural areas should ideally have separate sentinels, and a sentinel should represent only other districts that are assessed to have similar ecological, geographic, demographic, epidemiological, and socioeconomic characteristics.

> DSS is a system that has come to play a key role in health planning, not just in Tanzania but increasingly throughout the developing world.

Collecting, compiling, and updating population data is a massive task. This is clearly the case at the Rufiji DSS station at Ikwiriri, where station manager Dr E.A. Mwageni recently noted that he hasn't had a "computer-free day" since February 1999. The station is a beehive of activity throughout the week, often including weekends. As the nerve centre of health impact research taking place locally, the station houses the administrators and data processors who input the continuously updated health information that flows in from the field. Station personnel are fed this information from bicycle-equipped enumerators who travel to villages and households to update recent household characteristics and events. These local enumerators are responsible for two facets of data gathering: first, the collection of baseline data on precoded forms and, second, returning to every household every 4 months to update this information. "Key informants" — leaders in the community — preinform the enumerators when major changes (such as deaths) have occurred in the community (see box: "The growth of DSS monitoring").

Verbal autopsies

In cases where there has been a death in a household, specially trained interviewers are sent to conduct "verbal autopsies." These workers visit a household 2 to 4 weeks after a death has occurred. Deaths are also recorded in the system from biweekly visits to about 150 community key informants. Because of the sensitivity required when collecting information from bereaved families, conducting verbal autopsies is the sole task of these specialists. The autopsies follow a standardized international format and take several hours to complete. The advantage of a thorough interview — rich in context and detail — is that it minimizes the chance of misdiagnosis. In cases where symptoms, such as fever, could be caused by a number of underlying conditions, the contextual information could help point to the cause of death more precisely. Regardless, rates of accuracy will vary. However, statistical analysis confirms that, despite individual variations, in aggregate, verbal autopsies provide an accurate reflection of rates of disease within the general population. Causes of death are then assigned by a panel of three independent physicians.

On the web

THE RESEARCH

The growth of DSS monitoring

Since the first Demographic Surveillance System (DSS) was established in Bangladesh in the 1960s, the concept has grown as an international force to the point where DSS data is now gathered from large populations in approximately 30 locations in Africa. In 1998, the INDEPTH Network (an umbrella organization embracing 40 field sites in Africa, Southeast Asia, and Oceania) was constituted in a conference hosted by TEHIP and other Tanzanian DSS supporters in Dar es Salaam in 1998 to facilitate standardization and to promote evidence-based planning and the sharing of demographic information across borders. Increasingly, DSS is seen as essential not just in gathering and compiling household-level information on health, but also for monitoring trends related to poverty-reduction strategies, education, food security, and the environment.

The evolution of the tools

The DHMTs needed practical tools allowing them to easily understand information on local causes of mortality — the information that was collected through the DSS — and to incorporate that information into the health budgeting process. Exactly what tools would be needed, however, was not clear at the outset. Rather, new tools were developed intermittently over a 4- to 5-year period, as research pointed to gaps in the health planning process and as DHMTs identified areas where technical assistance was required.

What was known from the beginning, however, was that managers' practical requirements were different from the demands of the academic demographers and epidemiologists who had the time and training to sift through stacks of statistical charts and tables and to interpret the numbers. District planners — already burdened with excessive amounts of paper, statistics, and responsibilities — needed tools that could be integrated into their existing schedules and that would simplify and streamline their ongoing tasks, rather than add complexity to their routines.

The tools were therefore designed to give planners a quick overview of what bearing local health indicators had on budgeting and planning priorities. Information presented by the tools is invariably expressed in graphical form. Colourful charts and graphs allow managers to compare information easily and quickly and are much more readily understood than tables of numbers. The idea behind these tools was to empower district officials to deal with local needs. Said Morogoro District Executive Director John Gille: "The knowledge and skills we have acquired as a team have propelled us to a level whereby we can identify our problems, analyze our priorities, and construct an evidence-based plan." In addition, since local managers were integrally involved in developing the tools — by identifying gaps in the budgeting process and by helping to perfect those tools through use and experience — there was less risk than might otherwise exist that the tools would be rejected as "foreign" impositions and therefore not used.

Another test of how fully the tools could be integrated into planners' routines was whether they could perform more than one function. District planners are more likely to use a tool if it can help them to solve a variety of routine problems. By contrast, having individual, discreet tools that are brought out to solve individual problems represents extra work and distraction for busy managers. In this respect, the tools can be more aptly compared to a Swiss army knife than to a hammer or a saw. Both the burden of disease profile tool and the budget-mapping tool (1 and 2 below) serve about 10 routine, minor functions in addition to the main task they were designed to accomplish. They continue to evolve with time, experience, and use.

> District planners are more likely to use a tool if it can help them to solve a variety of routine problems.

On the web
THE RESEARCH

1. District burden of disease profile tool

This tool's primary job is to repackage population health information from the DSS in a way that district officials can easily understand. It provides an annual feedback at the start of the annual planning cycle on the population's health status and, consequently, its needs in terms of health interventions. This has led to planning revolutions in the two districts. District managers now have the means to set priorities during their planning that directly address the local burden of disease.

"Before TEHIP we did not identify and prioritize our interventions," recalls Dr Harun Machibya, Morogoro District Medical Officer. "Rather, we implemented plans worked out centrally. Even in budgeting, the tendency was to add some percentages to previous years' planned and budgeted activities." Peter Nkulila, a clinical officer on the DHMT concurs: "We did things blindly."

Not knowing how allocated resources corresponded to the local causes of mortality led to waste: for example, nonmalarious highland areas might receive (through a centrally planned process) a full allotment of antimalarial drugs more appropriate for an endemic area.

The burden of disease tool has allowed local officials to correct such problems by supplying them with information in a form that makes practical sense. Although a DSS had been operating and collecting data on the burden of disease in Morogoro since 1992, this information was not fully used by district health planners until the tools were introduced in 1997.

> Not knowing how allocated resources corresponded to the local causes of mortality led to waste.

Instead of unwieldy books of charts and numbers, the tool offers simple, computer-generated graphical representations of key indicators. These are known collectively as the "burden of disease profile." This profile is updated using the same sentinel DSS and distributed to all the district planners each year at a time corresponding to the district health planning period.

This tool is highly practical because it expresses burden of disease information in terms of "intervention addressable shares." Instead of presenting the burden of disease by specific disease categories, the profile shows the proportional burden addressed by various health interventions and strategies. These cost-effective interventions form a "package" of choices available to DHMTs. This is really a "district health intervention profile" and is more relevant to district planners — making it possible to appreciate the burden of disease in the context of health intervention priorities and the proportional use of resources to support such interventions. The tool also provides graphical representations of data on the age and seasonal distribution of deaths in the districts; place of birth or death; and health-seeking behaviour in the events preceding death. And since Tanzania has no vital statistics registry and national censuses are infrequent, the tool's provision of updated projections of population structure such as age and sex, current fertility, and age-specific mortality rates can help planners predict the number of births, deaths, infants, under-fives, pregnancies, and so on in the district in the next planning year. In turn, this can help guide the allocation of resources.

2. District health accounts tool

Also known as the "district health expenditures mapping tool," this software tool analyses budgets in a standard way to generate graphics that show how plans for spending — or current spending commitments — coalesce as a complete plan. Planners consulting these graphs are able to see how individual spending options translate as a proportion of their overall budget, where budget funding is coming from, and which interventions and activities are being funded.

On the web
THE RESEARCH

The tool is issued annually on diskette at the start of the district planning cycle. Planners input budget figures — representing the funding they want to allot to particular spending areas — into a matrix of standard line items and funding sources. The computer generates graphs illustrating the overall budgetary picture that would emerge from these inputs. One of the major advantages of this tool is that it reduces the complexity and extraneous details that often make it difficult for planners to keep track of where, proportionally, their funding is coming from and where it is going. Typically, district budgets provide multiple pages of detail and contain over a thousand budgeted items and activities, with hundreds of subtotals and dozens of major line items. Not only is it difficult to discern trends within this over-abundance of infor-mation, it is also difficult to spot errors and to make changes that will correct problems without creating new ones. The tool allows for changes to be made and then instantly generates the graphics showing how those changes will affect other aspects of the budget.

The tool also addresses a number of weaknesses that have emerged in the government–donor approach to health basket funding. As figures are entered, the tool checks the inputs against the ministry's expectations. If key issues have been left out or ceilings have been exceeded, for instance, the tool will bring this to the attention of planners. In several ways, this tool helps to ensure that budgets are not going to be rejected because they are noncompliant — any errors become readily apparent when the graphs are generated. The graphics also serve as important communication focal points in discussing the plan with stakeholders. DHMTs can also compare and contrast each other's annual plans from year to year.

3. District health service mapping tool

This tool uses a statistical database produced by the Health Management Information System in combination with an extensive catalogue of maps. The maps and the database are cross-referenced through a public domain tool developed by WHO called HealthMapper, a free software application, which was installed on all health planners' computers in Rufiji and Morogoro districts in June 2001.

The core function of the tool is to allow health administrators to use only a few keystrokes to get a quick, visual representation of the availability of specific health services or the attendance at health facilities for various diseases across the district. Maps provide detail down to the village level, showing roads, rivers, villages, administrative boundaries, health facilities, and schools. Those maps can in turn be overlaid by information depicting, for example, the immunization coverage in that particular area, the degree of malaria risk, and so on. Since human beings are inherently spatial and territorial, this mapped-out representation of the distribution of health indicators has a more visceral and direct impact on the reader than tables containing numbers and listings.

4. Community voice tool

"The lifeblood of the health sector reform is community participation," said Rufiji District Executive Director Faustin Fissoo.
"Using their own resources, communities have actively involved
themselves in initiating, planning, and managing their development projects." Noting some
villages' initial skepticism about
the idea that communities could
make strides without leadership
from upper levels of government,
Mr Fissoo relates that the community participation tool has
unleashed a new civic enthusiasm, which has had many practical
benefits. These range from the rehabilitation of village clinics
to the realization of numerous goals generated by community
members themselves.

> The lifeblood of the health sector
> reform is community participation.
> — Faustin Fissoo

On the web
THE RESEARCH

The community voice tool was introduced in recognition of the
value of communities expressing their own needs and wishes and
participating in bringing these goals to fruition. Sometimes these
communities' wishes are directly related to health care. Other
times, the communities identify their primary concerns as areas
indirectly connected with health (water supply, the condition of
roads, schooling, etc.).

Using an approach known as participatory action research,
animators have offered communities the opportunity to reflect on
their development preferences, pro-
moted dialogue on ways of achieving local participation in planning,
and identified individuals and
groups who can advance community participation. When communities are directly involved in
identifying and solving their own problems, community members
become a powerful force in programs of social improvement.

> When communities are directly
> involved in identifying and solving
> their own problems, community
> members become a powerful force
> in programs of social improvement.

For example, in Rufiji's Kilimani village, elders decided to raise money through a tax on local products such as cashews, rice, fish, and timber. The new funds have allowed Kilimani to provide piped water to the community. This has had multiple benefits: not only do many residents now have showers in their homes, but there has also been a reduction in the number of women injured by crocodiles since they no longer bring their laundry to the river bank. In Bungu, meanwhile, the community has built a new dispensary to replace a dilapidated one and has formed a women's group that has taken on projects such as making bricks to build a new school.

There is no proviso that strictly limits the use of the community voice tool to the health sphere. Indeed, one unexpected consequence of these activities has been that, once communities have been mobilized to express themselves on health care planning, the focus of community discussion often shifts to broader governance issues and to other matters such as the state of schools and roads. When community voice does focus directly on health issues, it sometimes facilitates an expression of community concerns (such as the provision of dental services and of first aid for skin conditions) that are more related to "quality of life" than to the mortality rate. Community voice also sometimes promotes discussion of how the health system can provide better service and what community members can do to improve their own health.

5. Cost-effectiveness and district cost information system tool

This is the "tool that got away." Understanding the incremental cost-effectiveness of health interventions was originally conceived of as one of the most important tools in the planning toolbox. It became apparent that two vital ingredients for cost-effectiveness analysis — costs and coverage — were not available to district planners. So the first step was to develop a cost-tracking tool. A very practical district-level computer database was developed to capture facility-specific intervention costs from a bottom-up approach. However, it found very little variance in costs between facilities or over seasons so it did not appear practical to run it continuously. It therefore stands as a useful tool to apply periodically to estimate the actual costs of interventions. As a research tool it was very useful to understand general technical inefficiencies and noncompliances. Districts still lack practical tools to estimate actual coverage of essential health interventions (with the exception of immunization and antenatal care where denominators are known). Without such developments, incremental cost-effectiveness considerations for decentralized planners are not possible, and planners are restricted to general information regarding generic cost-effectiveness from other settings.

Moving to the next stage

The tools have provided significant support to districts attempting to reform the way they plan to meet health challenges. The introduction of these tools coincided with two other developments that greatly strengthened the districts' abilities to plan health care delivery in line with the local disease burden: a budgetary top-up that brought health spending closer to the level recommended by WDR93 and a series of "supportive interventions and strategies"' designed to improve the efficiency of health care administration in Rufiji and Morogoro. The next chapter explores in greater detail how districts have used these tools and interventions to redesign and improve health care delivery.

Chapter 3

The Results

Women cradling babies sit along wooden benches outside the health clinic in Mvomero, a small rural community in Morogoro district. Inside, Mr Y.E. Kapito gently examines a baby to determine why he has a fever and to assess other health problems. The practitioner's quick reference guides are algorithmic, coloured wall charts that describe childhood illnesses, classification, and pathways to appropriate treatments.

Mr Kapito is seeing more patients these days. He estimates that the number has almost doubled in a year. But he hears of fewer child deaths. "It's been 6 to 8 months since I have heard about a child dying," he says. Samuel Hassain, who brought in his flu-stricken grandson, remarks, "Things have improved. People have faith in the services. They are treated well and get diagnosed properly."

Mvomero is one of many locations in Tanzania where the encouraging statistics showing lower mortality rates (particularly among children) take on a tangible form and a human face. It is here on the front lines — that critical arena where theory meets practice — where the reforms adopted by district health managers are proven either useful or ineffective.

One of the reasons why more children who come to the Mvomero clinic survive is that practitioners like Mr Kapito are now using a system called the Integrated Management of Childhood Illnesses (IMCI), one aspect of which is the use of those coloured charts. But such changes at the community level have also been accompanied — and, in fact, made possible by — some fundamental shifts in the way the health systems of Morogoro and Rufiji operate.

Essentially, improvements in the quality of health care have been the result of two factors. One is how district managers chose to use the planning tools; that is, what health interventions they decided to fund and prioritize in response to the portrait of burden of disease produced by the tools. DHMTs used these tools to overhaul the ways they planned, to revise their proportional allotment of funds, and to promote integrated solutions that offered multiple benefits from single health interventions.

The other key factor that allowed change to take place in the field was the availability of so-called "supportive interventions." Intended to restore some of the functional capacity that the health systems had lost because of years of under-funding and inertia, these interventions depended on districts' use of supplementary funding they had received from TEHIP. Both the use of the tools and the districts' investment in "supportive interventions" are examples of capacity building. However, they differ from each other in one key respect. The deployment of the tools is a form of **passive** capacity building: those tools didn't directly lead to change, but rather were one contribution that helped the districts enhance their own capacity to plan. The districts' provision of supportive interventions, on the other hand, is a more traditional form of capacity building that relies upon a direct transfer of skills through means such as training courses and targeted funding.

Supplementary funding

None of the changes to the ways that managers and clinicians go about their daily business would have happened without the provision of a modest financial top-up in the form of stakeholder funds to the districts. This new inflow of cash catalyzed an improvement of health care delivery by giving districts the financial means to act on their plans. These funds allowed districts to achieve new efficiencies in the daily operations of health systems and to increase spending where needed on interventions aimed at the most significant contributors to the local burden of disease.

The project first offered additional funding of up to US $2 per capita to the districts of Morogoro Rural and Rufiji in 1997. Surprisingly, however, both districts soon discovered that they were unable to absorb and spend this amount of extra funding. The $2 remained on offer for each of the first 3 years of the project. Still the districts did not have the capacity to absorb that amount of money. In 1997/98, 1998/99, and 1999/2000, the respective per capita consumption from the fund was US $0.57, $0.89, and $1.37. At this point, to spread the unspent money over a more reasonable period, the project was extended for 3 more years and the amount offered was reduced as the new national SWAp "basket" of US $0.50 per capita came into being (see box: "SWAp basket brings funding stability"). The average fund consumption over the first 4 years of the project was a US $0.92 annual per capita top-up contribution

> The health advances experienced in Rufiji and Morogoro were achieved at a per capita annual cost less than what someone in North America would pay for a cup of coffee.

SWAp basket brings funding stability

The SWAp district council health basket funds — consisting of resources received from a range of international development agencies active in the health sector in Tanzania — is administered by the Ministry of Health and made available to all districts of the country. The phasing in of the SWAp basket between 2001 and 2003 has addressed the difficult issue of the sustainability of top-up funding in the two districts as TEHIP has been phased out. Its creation has helped to ensure that the benefits that came with TEHIP top-up funding will remain as long as this new basket stays in place.

for the two districts. Expressed another way, the health advances experienced in Rufiji and Morogoro were achieved at a per capita annual cost less than what someone in North America would pay for a cup of coffee.

These extra funds were used by district planners to support essential health interventions, the rehabilitation of health facilities, and training and capacity-building activities, as well as to assist with the purchase of essential drug supplies, transportation, communications equipment, and computers and computer software. Ceilings were placed on the amount of funds that could be spent for health facility rehabilitation. The only other caveat was that intervention spending had to be consistent with evidence about the burden of disease and had to support only interventions known to be cost effective.

The districts' initial lack of capacity to absorb the additional US $2 in funding was at first baffling to the DHMTs. Why were the new funds sitting unused in a bank account? The answer was that health systems in Rufiji and Morogoro lacked the administrative and management capacity to put the funds to work. To absorb the top-up funding would have required the skill base to transform financial resources into program spending. Staff would have needed the skills enabling them to draw up contracts, hold structured meetings, issue cheques, procure supplies, interact with accountants, etc. – to do all the little things that are crucial to the functioning of a health system.

Capacity building in management and administration

The DHMTs saw in the mystery of the unspent funds a clue as to where they should invest a portion of the new money. It became clear that, for the system to be able to expand its budgets and service levels in the future, essential training and capacity building had to take place. Therefore, the DHMTs took stock of the missing skills and subsequently made use of a range of "supportive interventions" to address local deficits in management, administrative, and other skills.

For example, they acquired a modular training course called *Strengthening Health Management in Districts and Provinces,* developed by WHO (Cassels and Janovsky 1995), as a way of building the teams and increasing the confidence and skills of health management personnel. The basket funds also opened the space for the districts to purchase skills training for planners based on *Ten Steps to a District Health Plan*. Distributed by the Tanzanian Ministry of Health, the guide was developed by the Iringa Primary Health Care Institute (1997) in collaboration with the Nijmegen Institute for International Health.

This type of capacity building was crucial to the functioning of the DHMTs. Although the transfer of responsibility from high-level planners to locally based management teams was seen as central to Tanzania's health reforms, it was by no means assured that the team approach would succeed. Effective teams do not suddenly spring into existence – they need cultivation to acquire essential tools and skills and to develop over time. Trust and cooperation between members must be fostered, specialties must combine in ways that complement each other, and teams must learn how to delegate responsibility. And as the team approach moved outward to encompass facility staff and, indeed, whole communities (which participated in health reforms by helping to renovate health centres) so too did the list of partners needing training and capacity building expand.

In addition to management and team-strengthening courses, the new funds allowed the districts to pay for other supplemental capacity building and training that responded to perceived needs in a number of areas, including

➤ Report writing (quarterly, technical, and financial);

➤ Computer applications and training;

➤ Administrative and financial procedures (including financial management, inventory control, payment, and ledger maintenance);

➤ Office management (including components of office management such as filing, communication, email, appropriate channeling of communications, and organization of meetings, including writing of minutes, determination of action items, and delegation of tasks); and

➤ Regular maintenance of vehicles, radios, computers, health equipment, capital items, solar power, etc. Maintenance was largely overlooked in Tanzania, where capital goods and infrastructure would typically break or wear out ahead of schedule. Ensuring that costly items would last longer — because of regular maintenance — was essential to increasing the cost-effectiveness of the health system.

The Integrated Management Cascade

A large part of the work leading to the improved routine functioning of the district health systems was bundled together into a strategy known as the Integrated Management Cascade (IMC).

Focused largely on increasing capacity for the downward delegation of administrative duties to community-level workers (so that
those workers became more engaged in the process of improving
health care delivery), IMC was
designed to ensure the smooth
operation of the health system by
improving the links between community health workers and supervisory personnel. These links led to
greatly improved quality in the
health system by reducing prob-
lems that had existed in numerous areas, such as delivery of
drugs and supplies, distribution of staff pay, and the supervision
of health workers dealing with expenditures and the referral of
emergencies. All have major effects on the delivery of service.

> The Integrated Management Cascade
> was designed to ensure the smooth
> operation of the health system
> by improving the links between
> community health workers and
> supervisory personnel.

On the web
THE RESEARCH

Putting supervisors and workers in closer contact required innovations in transportation and communication — requirements
made all the more urgent by the challenging terrain of both Rufiji
and Morogoro. In Morogoro, the mountainous landscape makes
it difficult to travel between the district headquarters and out-
lying health facilities. The same is true for the Rufiji River delta
as well as the low-lying areas of the Rufiji flood plain, which are
rendered impassible during the rainy season when the river can
become a kilometres-wide torrent. Between March and May, the
rains wash away sections of road, making many facilities inacces-
sible. Moving between locations therefore comes at a high price:
finding alternative routes sometimes increases the distance three-
fold, leading to much greater use of fuel and staff time.

The solution? Districts used their top-up funding to equip each
health centre with a solar-powered radio (a model that was
robust and easy to operate) and to purchase a motorcycle, allowing supervisory personnel to travel quickly and cheaply between
facilities. Rufiji also invested some of its funding in a high-speed
boat to travel to villages in its vast tidal delta, since — in addition

to the problems of the rainy season — such health facilities are normally accessible only by water at high tide.

These modest investments in appropriate-scale transportation and communications technologies have improved workers' abilities to perform their daily duties. "We have a motorcycle in each facility that enables us to make supervision tours to our satellite dispensaries," says J.R. Lifa, Clinical Officer-in-Charge of Mgeta Rural Health Centre in Morogoro. "We also have radio equipment in each health centre, which facilitates easier communication between zones and the DHMT office."

Mr Amadeus Mwananziche, in charge at the Mlali Dispensary, says that the enhanced communication has improved functions ranging from delivery of drugs to referral of cases. "We can now inform each other when there is an epidemic and it is a lot easier to learn of any problems anywhere within my area of operation."

The new transportation and communication capacity has also made it possible to establish a better organizational structure known as the cascade management system. Previously, a core of 4 or 5 managers in a central office directly supervised 50 to 100 facilities — an almost impossible task, given the expectation that supervisors visit each dispensary 3 times a year. Now, supervisory responsibility "cascades" from staff in the central office to a secondary level of staff in the health centres. In turn they supervise a tertiary level of staff in the dispensaries within a reasonable traveling distance. This cascade structure, as depicted in Figure 2, has helped spread the benefits of new investments across the districts. Although labs and back-up drug supplies, for example, have been placed only in larger health centres, the use of radios and efficient means of transport have meant that clients who use smaller facilities can also share in the benefit of those investments.

Giving supervisors the physical means to oversee facilities within a more reasonable range has made it easier to solve routine problems. "We now have access to a working radio as well as email,"

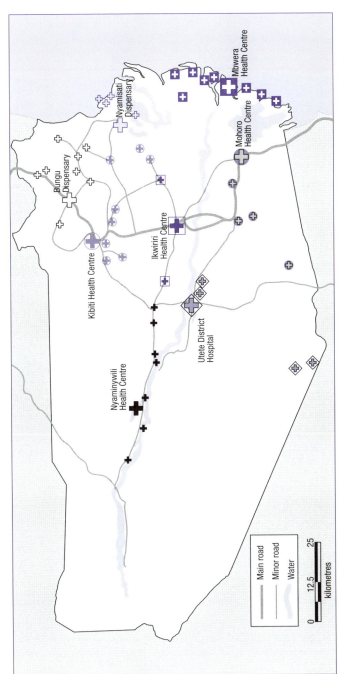

Figure 2. The management cascade. Supervision is delegated to staff at selected health facilities. This map shows the cascade system for Rufiji district. Facilities of the same colour and symbol are grouped together.

explains Dr Harun Machibya, Morogoro Rural District Medical Officer. "A simple matter that can now be solved by radio communication would have previously meant an officer boarding a bus to Dar es Salaam." To date, the management cascade has produced many positive results:

- Actual supervision of peripheral facilities with time for supervisors to directly observe patient care;
- More coherent laboratory specimen collection and diagnostic laboratory reporting functions;
- Timely delivery of drugs, equipment, and supplies;
- Coordination of referrals of patients to the district hospital;
- Emergency epidemic support, such as during cholera outbreaks;
- Routine collection of health information and data;
- Notification of arrival of staff salaries (resulting in reduced closure of health facilities as health workers travel to collect salaries too soon and have to wait before returning);
- Improved maintenance of facilities and equipment, and replenishment of stationary, registers, etc.;
- Improved linkages and communication with communities;
- Locally conducted capacity-building workshops, technical training, and refresher courses; and
- Posting of replacement health staff when regular personnel are ill or have died.

Instantaneous communication by radio has also had an uplifting impact on morale: community health workers can now be assured that help is on the way, rather than remaining uncertain about when district supervisors will respond to their inquiries or requests.

Rehabilitation of health facilities

At a spectacular ceremony at the Hanga Dispensary in Rufiji, the village chairperson walks from the audience to the podium, greets the area's member of parliament and returns to her seat holding a certificate signifying that members of the community now own their health facility. This effectively makes community members partners with upper levels of government in the provision of health care.

All across Rufiji and Morogoro, communities have entered into the same unique arrangement. The government has agreed to pay the salaries of health workers in the community and for drugs and supplies. In exchange, communities plan and contribute to the renovation of the local clinic with their inputs (such as local building materials) and labour, and pledge to maintain and run the facility. This citizen participation — part of a shift in emphasis away from central government toward local communities — is described by Dr Harun Machibya as "a breakthrough." Says Dr Machibya, "Before, people asked for help [from the government] even when a lock was broken."

This new partnership answers a crying need in the districts. Over the years, communities and Ministry of Health officials have expressed a consistent desire to see health facilities renovated. Built in the 1960s and 70s, village dispensaries had been neglected for several decades and many of them were dilapidated. Early on, a small amount of money available through TEHIP was set aside to study renovation options. A Ministry of Health architect was contracted to conduct a needs assessment that would gauge the state of each facility and rank them in order of priority. Photographs were taken of each facility and the numerous deficiencies of each were catalogued — a truly colossal task given that there were over 90 health facilities in Morogoro alone, demanding vast expenditures of time and energy.

It was soon clear that raising the necessary funds to renovate all these facilities would be impossible. But the Tanzanian "self-help" tradition from the postindependence period suggested a solution: what if officials asked communities to provide labour and some materials to offset the costs of renovation? A Tanzanian team familiar with community labour-based approaches was engaged to facilitate an initial demonstration exercise in 3 communities within each of the 2 districts. Community members were engaged in dialogue and work plans were produced. Rehabilitation of dispensaries in those communities took roughly 6 months. The communities' contribution of materials and labour meant that the renovation projects cost between 31% and 48% less than they would have cost under normal subcontracting practices.

Since then, this process has taken place in close to 40 communities. Some communities have gone well beyond what was in the standard dispensary blueprint by providing the health facilities with better latrines, water supply, and even extra maternity facilities. In some cases, the momentum from health facility rehabilitation has spurred other changes, with community members initiating new upgrading projects for mosques, schools, health workers' houses, and other local amenities.

The celebrations that invariably accompany completion of the health facility renovations provide an opportunity not just for revelry but also for government representatives to acknowledge the citizens' contribution. In Lusanga, for instance, as members of the community and the DHMT gathered in a carnival atmosphere, a high-ranking official presented a gift to the community. This gift took the form of more than 2 million Tanzanian shillings (US $1 800 in July 2004) worth of health equipment, including in-patient and delivery beds, suction equipment, and a blood pressure machine. Ownership of the building was then transferred to the community — a gesture that stands as a reverse image of what occurred 30 to 40 years earlier, when communities transferred ownership of health facilities they had built to the central government.

What the districts did with budget planning tools

In addition to the "supportive interventions," other reforms —
aimed at changing how community health workers dealt with
disease — took place on a parallel track. Health managers at the
district level, newly equipped with the planning tools, began
restructuring health services to focus resources on the greatest
need. Armed with new and current knowledge about the burden

THE RESEARCH

What the research revealed

Research into three distinct areas — health systems, health behaviour, and
health impacts — provided critical insights that aided health care reforms in
Rufiji and Morogoro. One of the most striking findings of the inquiries into
health-seeking behaviours, for example, was that most deaths (close to
80%) occurred at home rather than at a health facility. This statistic underscored earlier doubts about the use of attendance and cause-of-death
statistics — compiled by the government on the basis of health facility data
only — as an aid for planning health budgets. Surely, this form of planning
could not be reliable since it was based on only 20% of deaths. Since DSS
information, by contrast, captures all deaths — those that occur in health
facilities, in households, and elsewhere — it can be counted upon to give a
more accurate and complete portrait of the burden of disease as experienced by the community.

Another surprising revelation arising from research into health-seeking
behaviour was that the people who had sought modern health care prior to
their deaths greatly outnumbered those who had not. As illustrated in Figure 3,
for malaria, 78.7% used modern care, only 9.4% used traditional care, and
11.9% used no care at all. These figures prove that the death rates in Rufiji
and Morogoro were not primarily an outgrowth of a preference for traditional
healers over modern health care (as some observers had speculated), but
are more reasonably seen as related to problems of access, delay, or the
apparent inability of modern health facilities to prevent these patients from
dying. Formative research into the health systems planning process confirmed that planning was not being conducted as a response to the burden
of disease, but instead was driven by a wide range of factors including
donor agencies' agendas, bureaucratic inertia, and simple guesswork.

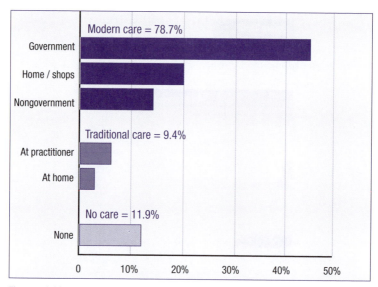

Figure 3. Initial care-seeking patterns. Care of first resort sought during the final illness by 320 fatal malaria cases in children less than 5 years of age in the Rufiji DSS sentinel area, 1999–2001. (Source: de Savigny et al. 2004)

of disease in their district — and with tools that allowed them to track spending in line with that burden of disease — these managers tried to ensure that spending on individual health services would provide a significant pay-off in terms of lives saved and illness prevented. Districts also had new insight into the ways the health system could be improved since they had access to the results of research undertaken by the research consortia (see box: "What the research revealed").

What did burden of disease profiles and budget analysis tools tell district managers? Figure 4 provides some indications of how the actual local burden of disease corresponded to recent health care spending. In Morogoro district, for example, spending on malaria had been significantly lower than would have been expected for an illness that was the single biggest cause of mortality in the district. Following the introduction of the planning tools and additional funding, Morogoro's proportional expenditures came

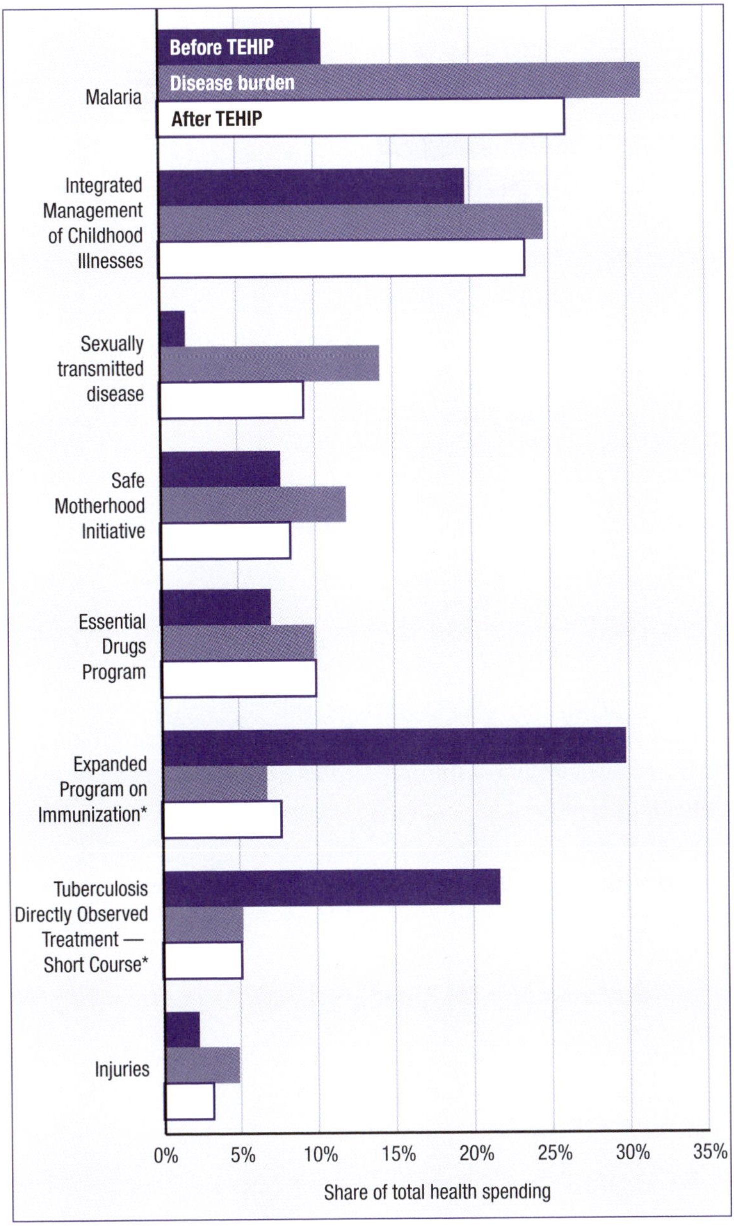
Before TEHIP
Disease burden
After TEHIP
Malaria
Integrated Management of Childhood Illnesses
Sexually transmitted disease
Safe Motherhood Initiative
Essential Drugs Program
Expanded Program on Immunization*
Tuberculosis Directly Observed Treatment — Short Course*
Injuries
0%
5%
10%
15%
20%
25%
30%
35%
Share of total health spending

Figure 4. Morogoro district health spending before (1996/97) and after (2000/01) the introduction of TEHIP budget mapping tool.

* Absolute funding levels for immunization and tuberculosis remained unchanged while funding for other interventions increased.

more into line with its burden of disease. Meanwhile, in districts where planning tools were not introduced, the imbalance remained striking.

Evidence provided by the DSS indicated to health planners that two areas in particular accounted for a huge proportion of the burden of disease: acute febrile illness (including malaria) and a cluster of diseases affecting young children (acute febrile illness, pneumonia, diarrhoea, malnutrition, anemia, and measles). While a few individual districts did provide reasonable funding for these illnesses, aggregate numbers for all of Tanzania show, in general, insufficient funding to fight the biggest killers. Nation-wide, childhood illnesses accounted for 37% of burden of disease: they received 17% of funding (Figure 5). A bigger problem is that the largest funding share (sometimes over 50%) went to a multitude of marginal problems with a cumulative burden of less than 15% (Figure 6).

One way that district managers could more effectively face the challenges posed by the real burden of disease was by paying close attention to what went into the "minimum package of interventions" to be used by community health workers. They could, in other words, make sure that every remedy was useful in the local context. Table 2 details what was included in this minimum package in Rufiji and Morogoro. Every intervention in the package had to address a significant portion of the burden of disease, either a single or collective illnesses or conditions that contributed at least 2% or more to the burden of disease or an eradicable condition.

A new assault on disease

District managers also ensured they had well thought-out programs in place to combat the conditions that accounted for very large shares of the burden of disease. Since the most burdensome conditions were malaria and illnesses of young children, health

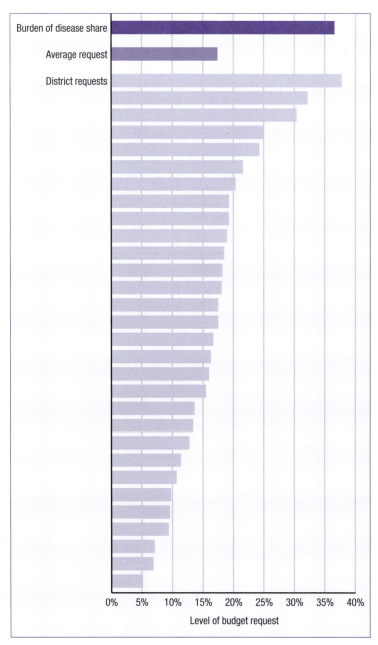

Figure 5. **Districts planning without tools: budget requests for IMCI in 30 district health plans, 2002.**

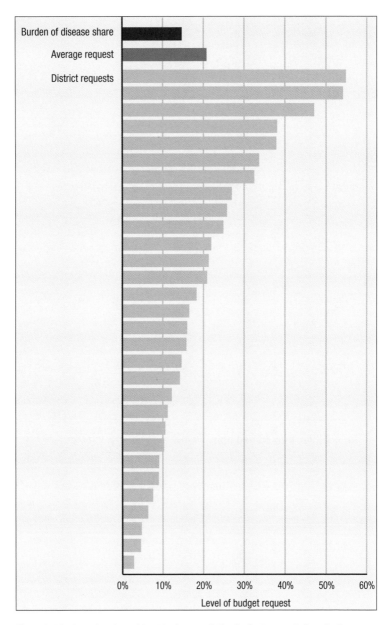

Figure 6. Districts planning without tools: cumulative budget requests for all other interventions, each of which individually address less than 1% of the total burden of disease in 30 district health plans, 2002.

managers put a heavy emphasis on malaria control and the Integrated Management of Childhood Illnesses (IMCI).

Malaria is a disease that already had been identified at the national level as a huge threat to public health. In the wake of daunting evidence that conventional drug therapies for malaria were failing, the Ministry of Health had embarked on a new antimalarial drug policy using a newer drug. The Ministry has also been involved in the promotion of insecticide-treated bed nets, which are deemed particularly vital in protecting pregnant women and babies from the devastating effects of malaria infection. TEHIP and its tools have fed into the antimalaria assault at both the district and national levels. Locally, the tools showed managers that insufficient resources were being applied to combating malaria and persuaded them to reverse this trend. Nationally, the project's advice was sought in the development of new mechanisms to increase the distribution of bed nets across Tanzania (see box: "The need for treated bed nets").

It is important to note that there is a significant intersection between the two leading contributors to burden of disease: IMCI-addressable conditions and acute febrile illness (AFI).

The need for treated bed nets

Although the efficacy of insecticide-treated bed nets (ITNs) for preventing mortality was only established in 1996, the evidence in their favour is impressive. The Tanzanian Ifakara Health Research and Development Centre has determined that ITNs could prevent 30 000 deaths and more than 5 million clinical episodes of malaria annually in Tanzania. Research summarized in *Net Gain*, a copublication of IDRC and WHO, indicates that ITNs could reduce child mortality in Africa by at least 17% (Lengeler et al. 1996). Treated nets are also one of the most cost-effective ways of preventing death and illness. And their benefits appear to be community-wide rather than merely personal: recent evidence shows that an area with a high concentration of treated bed nets affords some protection for all people in that area, even those who do not own a bed net themselves. Treated bed nets were one of the selected essential health interventions in these evidence-driven districts.

Table 2. Tanzania's national package of essential health interventions

Reproductive and child health

• Safe motherhood: maternal conditions

> Intermittent presumptive treatment of malaria (pregnancy); antenatal care; obstetric care; postnatal care; gynaecology, STD, HIV/AIDS care; micronutrient supplementation for mothers

• Safe motherhood: perinatal conditions

> STD screening; support for traditional birth attendants; safe delivery practices; newborn care; micronutrient supplementation for low birth weight babies; village birth registers

• Immunization

> BCG (tuberculosis); diphtheria; pertussis; neonatal tetanus; measles; poliomyelitis; hepatitis B

• Integrated Management of Childhood Illnesses (IMCI)

> Malaria; pneumonia; diarrhoea; measles; malnutrition; anemia

• Family planning

• Nutritional deficiencies

> Nutrition information, education, and communication; breast-feeding support groups; growth monitoring and pupil health screening; micronutrient supplementation (iron, vitamin A); monitoring salt iodization; deworming; school feeding

Communicable disease control

• Malaria

> IMCI (early care seeking and case management); insecticide-treated bed nets; intermittent presumptive treatment in pregnancy; home-based care; school health education about malaria prevention; epidemic preparedness; sustainable source reduction; information, education, and communication

• Tuberculosis and leprosy

> Tuberculosis Directly Observed Treatment — Short Course (DOTS); leprosy multidrug therapy; home-based care

• HIV/AIDS and STDs

> STD prevention; information, education, and communication; condom promotion; blood screening; patient care, counseling, and social support; palliative care

• Epidemic preparedness

> Cholera, measles, meningitis, plague, and malaria

(continued)

Table 2. concluded

Noncommunicable disease control

- Cardiovascular diseases
    IEC on smoking, alcohol, diet, and exercise

- Diabetes
    Preventive and promotive IEC; routine checking of blood pressure

- Neoplasms
    Breast and cervical cancer screening

- Injuries and trauma care

- Mental disorders

- Anemia and nutritional deficiencies

Treatment for common diseases

- Helminths, skin, ocular, and oral conditions

Community health promotion and disease prevention

- School health

- Water hygiene and sanitation

- Information, education, and communication
    Seven interventions

Source: Ministry of Health, Tanzania. 2000. National package of essential health interventions in Tanzania. Government of Tanzania, Dar es Salaam, Tanzania. pp. 1–123.

Note: In the essential package, there are more than 50 technical interventions but not all have equal priority in different settings. STD, sexually transmitted disease; BCG, Bacillus Calmette-Guerin; IMCI, Integrated Management of Childhood Illnesses; IEC, information, education, and communication strategy.

AFI (including malaria) represents over 60% of IMCI-addressable conditions in Tanzania. Indeed, malaria is more debilitating for children than it is for adults and is a contributor to many child deaths that are not recognized as having been caused by malaria. Districts have therefore focused particularly on combating malaria infection in the very young (see box: "'Malaria's threat to the young").

On the web
THE RESEARCH

Malaria's threat to the young

Many adults may not intuitively recognize malaria as a deadly disease for children because their own experience of malaria may be quite different. Adults who have survived malaria earlier in life are not likely to later die from it. Although they may suffer regular episodes, they have developed partial immunity and can be more readily treated. For children, however, malaria is debilitating in a number of ways. After the first few months of life, a baby will lose the immune protection it has acquired passively from its mother and may experience acute fever, anemia, convulsions, and other dangerous complications as a result of malarial infection. The child will then enter a downward cycle where lack of appetite and constant stress will push him or her off the growth curve, suppress the immune system, and leave the child more vulnerable to other diseases. When the child becomes thoroughly debilitated from fighting the malaria parasites, the next experience of illness — be it diarrhoea or another episode of malaria — is more likely to be fatal.

Malaria is also directly responsible for many childhood deaths that masquerade as other illnesses. Since the malaria parasite multiplies in red blood cells — eventually causing the red blood cells to disintegrate, before moving on to inhabit other red blood cells — children with malaria exhibit acute anemia. Anemia in young African children is difficult for mothers and health workers to spot. A drop of blood from a child with severe anemia from malaria will often appear pale pink instead of red on a piece of blotter paper. This malaria-related anemia may set in motion a series of other tragic consequences. When the red blood cell count is low, it is difficult for oxygen to be transported through the blood stream. As a result, the child's heart is under enormous strain. Sometimes the result is sudden cardiac failure — an event that appears to parents and to many clinicians to be unrelated to malaria.

Integrated Management of Childhood Illnesses

The first adaptation and pretest (or trial) of the Integrated Management of Childhood Illnesses (IMCI) took place in Arusha, Tanzania, in February 1995. Since then, WHO and UNICEF have produced generic materials for this approach, and IMCI is now being implemented in many developing countries.

IMCI is a care strategy that takes a "syndromic" approach, addressing the whole child by identifying and treating a range of possible common illnesses rather than simply focusing on one disease at a time. The fact that sick children will present with symptoms that may be caused by a number of possible diseases — or that they may suffer several diseases at once, or have one condition masquerading as another — provides a strong case for this integrated approach.

> The fact that sick children will present with symptoms that may be caused by a number of possible diseases provides a strong case for this integrated approach.

On the web
THE RESEARCH

When district managers in Rufiji and Morogoro recognized and sought to lower childhood mortality rates, adopting IMCI became an obvious choice. Implementing the program, however, required major efforts: retraining front-line health workers, reorganizing the use of clinic space, and promoting and encouraging a more active health-seeking role and better skills for parents — all of which had to be addressed simultaneously.

Consider the fundamental shifts in practice that IMCI has required. Before IMCI, children brought by a parent to a clinic would be seen in a "factory line" process. The health worker might guess, for example, that the child's problem was diarrhoea and dispense a standard treatment. The process was one of quick evaluation and the rapid consumption of certain drugs. When districts sought to change this, they began with staff retraining. Groups of workers were taken out of the field and given a specific course of training and new bedside clinical instruction. When they returned to work, workers would be "validated"' to ensure that they had absorbed the new methods.

The differences in the way health workers are now expected to deal with patients start with the children's arrival at the clinic. Children are assessed to gain some sense of the seriousness of their condition. Patients exhibiting danger signs move to the front of the queue. To streamline the work, a clinic assistant takes care of simple processing such as taking temperatures and weights of patients in the queue. Today, a health worker examining a child is no longer expected to guess at the root cause of the child's ailment. Instead, the worker consults a set of algorithms: when certain signs and symptoms are present, the practitioner is guided to the possible causes of those symptoms and to the appropriate treatment and prescription. This is part of the "syndromic" approach — the health worker is prepared to accept that the child may be suffering from a series of conditions working in concert, rather than from one particular disease.

Health workers believe that major gains have been achieved from adopting this approach. "I am impressed with the achievements attending the under-fives," says Tarsis Bwakila, clinical officer at the Ikwiriri Health Centre. "The way of managing diseases has improved. A good indicator of improved services is the increasing number of patients coming to our facility."

Another key feature of IMCI is that the parent, normally the mother, is integrally involved in the process. After the practitioner explains the main causes of the child's condition to the parent, the first dose of the appropriate treatment is given by the parent at the clinic, under the observation of the health worker. The health worker is therefore certain that the parent knows how to use the drug. (Diagrammatic instructions are also sent home with the parent as a reminder of how and when treatment is to be administered.) The parent is then told about the importance of proper and continued feeding (including the provision of more fluids), danger signs, and what to do if the child does not improve. To verify the parent's understanding, he or she is asked to recount the danger signs and the actions to take when these signs appear or when the child does not get better. This is part of an attempt to improve awareness and health practices in the home.

The selection of drugs also supports the practice of "syndromic" classification. Rather than prescribe drug A, which works very well against condition X, or drug B, which works very well against disease Y, the health worker has been taught that it is better to prescribe drug C, which does a reasonable job of combating both diseases X and Y. In other words, the idea is to choose drugs that have a broader spectrum of coverage. The IMCI methodology has proven highly adaptable to situations where adequately trained clinicians are in short supply. Personnel with limited clinical training can perform very well using the IMCI system. Indeed, because the process is guided by algorithms, lower skill workers may stick to the IMCI program more rigorously than better trained professionals and be less likely to revert to the use of "intuition."

The results of this process have been dramatic. The introduction of IMCI corresponded to a significant increase in the quality of child health services and a reduction of child mortality rates in Rufiji and Morogoro districts. In Morogoro, child mortality between the late 1990s and early 2000s has declined over 40% — from about 35:1000 to around 20:1000 annual deaths in children under 5 years of age. An important share of this reduction has been shown to be the direct result of the IMCI system.

> The introduction of IMCI corresponded to a significant increase in quality of child health services and a lowering of the child mortality rates in the Rufiji and Morogoro districts.

In addition, there is reason to speculate that the corresponding lowering of adult mortality rates in those districts may also be related to improvements in skills brought about by the introduction of IMCI. Partly, this is likely the result of better health-seeking behaviour and patient attendance at facilities — as adults see better results for their children, they are more likely to seek health care for themselves. In addition, adults may benefit from better treatment. As practitioners who deal with children also deal with adults, it is logical to expect that health workers would apply some of the organizational and clinical skills they learned in IMCI to the treatment of older patients.

Amadeus Mwananziche, medical assistant in charge at Mlali Dispensary, agrees with that assumption. "The training we received in IMCI and other areas has helped us a great deal in the management of other diseases," he says. Instituting an adult version of integrated management of illness is something being considered by WHO as a future health intervention, given the success of the "child version."

The two districts' positive introduction and experience with IMCI also underscores the critical need for continual retraining and upgrading of staff. This, in fact, is just one of many lessons arising from the TEHIP experience, which are explored in the next chapter.

Conclusion

The multitude of program initiatives set in motion by TEHIP are wide-ranging but not scattered. They form a coherent whole that, we believe, has helped dramatically reduce infant, child, and adult mortalities in a population of approximately 741 000 (greater that the population of 66 of the world's countries). In short, the relationship between these seemingly disparate program elements can be summarized as follows:

Increased technical efficiency of the health system (through stronger planning, management, and administration at the district level)	+	Increased allocative efficiency of the health system (through prioritized selection of interventions and budgeting focused on the largest "intervention-addressable shares" of burden of disease)	+	New incremental funding with decentralized control	=	Higher quality and greater utilization of health services, and better population health

Chapter 4

Extending TEHIP's Innovations and Impact

One of the paradoxes emerging from a successful demonstration project — even one as wide in scope as TEHIP — is that once the program winds down, its work has only just begun. The project demonstrated some positive impact from the innovations it tested. Intensive follow-up, dissemination of findings, and promotion of new and successful approaches are needed.

Accomplishing those goals is neither simple nor easy. Yet fairness demands that innovations such as the tools, which have clearly helped to improve the mortality and burden of disease pictures in

Rufiji and Morogoro, must be made available to other districts within Tanzania and to other countries. That is why IDRC crafted an "exit strategy" designed to ensure that the management tools, supportive interventions, innovative practices, and new ideas generated during TEHIP's life will continue to flourish and improve the effectiveness of district health systems long after the project itself has ended.

> Fairness demands that innovations such as the tools must be made available to other districts within Tanzania and to other countries.

The work initiated by TEHIP can be seen as a two-stage process. The first stage was the development, testing, refinement, and trial use of the products and strategies during the lifespan of the project. The second phase is the promotion of these products and strategies more widely within the Ministry of Health and to the huge number of additional districts that have not yet benefited from their use.

It should be noted that — since the tools and strategies now exist — the second, "roll-out" phase is much less costly than the research and development phase that preceded it. No new research or development of new products is required at this stage; that would be "reinventing the wheel." Mostly, adapting the tools for use in other districts (and, indeed, other countries) depends on the provision of local data. That data is less difficult to produce than it might have been several years ago, since Demographic Surveillance Systems (DSSs) are increasingly used throughout the developing world. Another critical requirement for the "roll-out" phase is training: health planning teams and community-level health workers in other districts need to know what the tools can do for them and how to use them. Spreading new knowledge to various levels within the health system therefore requires the cultivation of new cadres of trainers — the agents of change who can communicate new methods and ideas to essential workers in communities and in district offices.

As TEHIP ends as a project, the second phase of work is well underway. The Ministry has taken ownership of the tools and innovations and, with international funding — primarily from the United Nations Foundation — is now laying the base for their use throughout Tanzania.

Some of the specific "roll-out" measures now underway are as follows:

→ Ministry of Health zonal training centres (ZTCs) are being strengthened and coordinated into a network capable of delivering quality curricula to health workers. These centres will provide continuing education to upgrade the skills of existing health workers and will train new workers. The workers will be trained in essential interventions such as IMCI and in new, forthcoming interventions that will address HIV/AIDS. In addition, ZTCs will be an important vehicle for rolling out the tools. For example, training in the community voice and the district health accounts tools is now being offered by ZTCs. Use of ZTCs to promote the tools throughout Tanzania will show that these tools are sustainable and can endure beyond TEHIP since their promotion to the remaining districts will be accomplished using local staff exclusively.

→ The United Nations Foundation (with administrative support from WHO) has funded the roll out of the entire tool kit to 11 other Tanzanian districts. Additionally, by August 2004, DHMTs in approximately half of the country had been trained in the use of the burden of disease profile and the district health accounts tools. It is hoped that

> The United Nations Foundation has funded the roll out of the entire tool kit to 11 other Tanzanian districts.

all districts will have those two essential planning tools by the start of the 2005 planning cycle. In addition, interest in the tools has been expressed outside of Tanzania. DANIDA (the Danish International Development Agency) has put the budget-mapping tool on extended trial; WHO is planning to test the same tool in Ghana; and the Rockefeller Foundation is interested in adapting it to Uganda. South Africa has also expressed a general interest in the TEHIP approach. Finally, the INDEPTH Network has been training DSS sites elsewhere in Africa and Asia in the use of the burden of disease profile tool.

➤ The management cascade and the manual to guide community-led rehabilitation of health facilities have been adopted by Tanzania's Ministry of Health. The cascade has been introduced to other districts and the Ministry is poised to do the same with the facility rehabilitation tool. Increasingly, the widespread benefits of these programs are being recognized at a national level within Tanzania. The cascade system, for instance, has been praised for its effectiveness in devolving responsibility to lower levels within the health system. It has thus had a positive impact on morale by providing new challenges and increased job satisfaction for workers in the communities. In addition, the cascade's impact in giving local communities greater access to lab diagnostics is seen as increasingly important as the country gears up for new responses to HIV/AIDS. Community rehabilitation of health facilities, meanwhile, has been embraced largely because of its sustainability, cost-effectiveness, and lack of reliance on specialized expertise.

Other ideas and strategies that were incorporated into plans created by Rufiji and Morogoro DHMTs — as a result of those teams' use of the planning tools and input — have captured the attention of planners at various levels. They will likely come into wider use, promising further improvement in health indicators. For example:

➤ IMCI — a strategy originally devised by WHO — became an obvious choice for district planners searching for cost-effective health interventions after the tools illustrated that a huge proportion of the local burden of disease resulted from a small, interconnected web of childhood illnesses. Once IMCI was adopted by districts and brought into practice through the funding top-up, its ancillary benefits became obvious. For one, IMCI — by encouraging the practitioner to look at the patient as a whole person rather than as merely the host for a particular disease — has in many cases increased the quality and sensitivity of care by returning the focus to the patient rather than the illness. For another, it soon became apparent that diagnosing and treating a wide range of (sometimes coexisting) illnesses was more cost-efficient than first imagined. Now, there are plans to expand the use of "integrated" treatment regimes to other illnesses. For example, WHO has led the development of the Integrated Management of Adolescent and Adult Illness (IMAI) program — the so-called "adult version" of IMCI. IMAI is now at an advanced stage. In addition, there is renewed interest in revising and updating similarly integrated maternal care programs.

> IMCI has in many cases increased the quality and sensitivity of care by returning the focus to the patient rather than the illness.

➤ Within Tanzania, the presence of TEHIP as a conduit for research to find its way into the health system — that is, its function of promoting research as an influence on health care planning and practice — has stimulated ideas about the need for a new mechanism to package and synthesize the best and most recent research for use by political decision-makers. IDRC has provided initial funding to investigate what form such a national-scale health policy "observatory" might take. This health research observatory has been tentatively named the "Duluti Institute" after a landmark meeting of health researchers and policymakers in Duluti, Arusha, Tanzania.

➤ Tanzania is extending the reach of Demographic Surveillance Systems (DSSs). The DSS in Rufiji is now being operated by the Ifakara Health Research and Development Centre, which also operates DSS sites in 2 other districts. The INDEPTH Network

On the web
THE LESSONS

promises more integrated work in demographic surveillance between countries.

Finally, it should be noted that TEHIP has never advocated a static approach to dealing with health care needs — instead, it has encouraged flexibility and responsiveness to changing conditions. Given the promise of a general improvement in the functioning of Tanzania's health system — an improvement for which TEHIP is partly responsible — we expect that health authorities will reassess their goals and approaches in reaction to changed circumstances. One such realignment already underway is the shift in emphasis from cost-effectiveness to a more specific concern with equity. With the promise that a greater segment of the population will have access to effective health care services, it has become incumbent upon officials to address the equity issue by examining how they can reach out to the remaining segments of society that haven't benefited from overall advances. One example of this is the government's new approach to allotting basket funding. It has been decided that districts where there is hardship will receive an "equity premium" — a per capita allowance that is slightly above the national average.

One way of understanding this "cost-effectiveness versus equity" issue is to think of the health system as a car. A few years ago, the entire system wasn't working well — the car was only firing on two cylinders and the tires were flat. The Rufiji and Morogoro cases demonstrated that taking an initial efficiency approach could get the car running again: well-targeted investments could produce good results that serve the majority of the population. But there is no reason to stop there. There are other health issues — such as equity — to be addressed. The question for society at large becomes: Now that the car is working again, where shall we go? This is a social policy question, rather than a technical one, that will need to be asked continually.

Chapter 5

Lessons Learned

*The way health systems are designed, managed and
financed affects people's lives and livelihoods. The
difference between a well-performing health system and
one that is failing can be measured in death, disability,
impoverishment, humiliation, and despair.*
— Gro Harlem Brundtland (WHO 2000)

The lowering of mortality rates and disease burden in Rufiji and
Morogoro supports the initial premise that TEHIP set out to test.
The burden of disease can be significantly lowered through relatively low-cost investments in strengthening health systems by
providing incremental, decentralized, sector-wide health basket
funding — and a tool kit of practical management, planning, and
priority-setting tools that assist an evidence-based approach. In
other words, **investing in health systems works**.

What else have we learned? During several years of intensive research and fieldwork, the TEHIP team has observed many situations that we feel are instructive for health system development. This chapter lists a few critical lessons arising from that experience. All relate to the task of strengthening health systems and are organized under the thematic categories of general principles, people, information, infrastructure, and governance. These are all crucial components to ensure the effective delivery of health care. Investing in these essential pillars of health care delivery will maximize any corollary gains achieved through the introduction of new drugs, treatments, and interventions.

General principles

A significant amount of new money needs to be dedicated to strengthening basic health systems in developing countries to allow the scaling-up of coverage of existing essential health interventions. Basic health services — widely distributed but tightly integrated — are the foundations upon which advances in health can be based.

Where possible, initiatives to improve health should take advantage of the synergies created by combining research and development functions into a mutually reinforcing, integrated system. Funding research and development activities simultaneously — and encouraging researchers and development specialists to be aware of and involved in each other's specific areas of concern — produces multiple benefits. Foremost among these is that important research findings can be acted upon quickly: there is no need to reapply for funding before the development stage can proceed. Also, development plans can benefit from continuous input from researchers: effectiveness can be

> Being linked to a concrete development agenda affords researchers greater credibility within communities.

monitored and improvements can be made as work proceeds. Finally, being linked to a concrete development agenda affords researchers greater credibility within communities.

People

Investments must be made to increase and improve human resources to implement health services. IMCI, the Integrated Management of Childhood Illnesses — a key expression of health reforms instituted in the districts — illustrates how crucial training and retraining are to success. In addition, projected population growth, workforce attrition, and changing patterns of disease indicate that major and continuing investments in human resources will be crucial if Africa is to meet the coming challenges. For example, models published by Kurowski et al. (2003) predict that in a country like Tanzania, even with large increases in training capacity, the work force available for the health sector will decrease by up to 25% by the year 2015.

Coming at a time when most health problems are increasingly preventable, when health threats and strain on health services are also expected to increase, and when significant new resources for health are being mobilized, these work force statistics highlight the need for a major increase in human resources for health. New expenditures should include funding for initial training, retraining, and continuing education, as well as for the development of new curricula to address and update health workers' knowledge of new interventions and guidelines.

Infrastructure

Significant amounts of money must be made available for the "bricks and mortar" aspects of health care — essential capital resources like community clinics, vehicles to transport providers and supplies to where they are needed, and information and communication technologies. The size of investments required will vary from country to country. While in Tanzania, a good network of health facilities was already in place (albeit, in various states of disrepair), such facilities may not exist in other countries.

> Significant amounts of money must be made available for the "bricks and mortar" aspects of health care.

Governance

Rather than depending on a series of remotely planned, disease- or intervention-specific programs, funding and implementation priorities must increasingly be based upon locally owned, evidence-based plans that aim to develop the health system, maximize health, and reduce inequities. Ministries of health, local government, and health system managers need to ensure that regulations and standards for quality of care and service delivery are adequately maintained.

Health-related project initiatives should be designed with an "exit strategy" in mind, so that local ownership and buy-in, sustainability, and momentum become factors that are likely to extend the influence of the project once the project managers have left. It is important to provide funding for the machinery — such as the training of local-level professional trainers — so that the benefits of a promising project will extend both nationally and internationally.

The benefits of health "observatories" must be recognized. It is here that current research can be assembled, packaged, and translated into accessible language so that governmental decision-makers in health are better equipped to do their jobs. Researchers cannot be expected to have the appropriate skills to disseminate their findings to politicians and government officials.

That task requires another level of specialists who will function as intermediaries between the research community and the architects of the health system.

Information

To optimize the use of limited financial resources, health spending must respect and encourage local evidence-based priorities rather than the agendas of donors and "vertical" programs. As experience with decentralization proceeds, it is no longer appropriate for districts in developing countries to be compelled to design their local budgets and programs around the priorities of bilateral and multilateral agencies. Additionally, it is advantageous to avoid competitive situations that can arise between international donors. The sector-wide approach (SWAp) — which pools international sectoral contributions to create a funding "basket" — is one example of how competition can be avoided and cooperation encouraged.

Furthermore, the availability of data through sentinel population-based information systems provides a disincentive for the continuation of vertical, sometimes competitive agendas promoted by single organizations. Donors and funders sometimes promote vertical initiatives because this is the easier way of monitoring the impact of their program spending. However, Demographic Surveillance System data can provide a measure of accountability by demonstrating whether, cumulatively, international contributions have had an impact on mortality rates.

In countries not yet able to afford or manage functional vital event registration of births, deaths, and causes of death — including most of sub-Saharan Africa — there should be an alternative of at least two (one rural, one urban) sentinel or sample Demographic Surveillance Systems. These would function as minimum, cost-effective population, health, and poverty observatories. More such sentinels are needed in countries with greater diversity in health risk patterns. DSSs should also be employed with a view to the integrated use of several different streams of information (such as health status, poverty indicators, and equity indicators), all of which flow from sentinel DSS monitoring. These systems can provide an important share of the evidence base for local planners.

If health-intervention systems are to play their role effectively as instruments for improving health, they must be designed to support the decisions and actions of health personnel. They may also be part of an integrated poverty-monitoring system. Health workers also need access to population-based information and to practical information on how to manage health facilities. This points, for example, to an urgent need to develop new tools to help district planners understand health service access and coverage, and where and how it fails. It also points to the importance of assisting the health system to scale up once its technical and allocative deficiencies have been addressed. Information must be presented to managers and management teams in an easily understood fashion. Local-level managers have neither the time nor the luxury of sifting through large amounts of data to determine what information is of practical use to them. Presenting such data precisely and graphically will speak to these managers in ways that allow them to make better, evidence-based decisions.

Conclusion

As the accounts contained in this book have shown, TEHIP has been largely concerned with assisting decentralized health system managers address technical and allocative inefficiencies by increasing their access to new management skills and new forms of local evidence. More work is required, however.

In the medium term, the challenge is to strengthen and consolidate the indigenous structures capable of absorbing the hard-won lessons of the district health managers in Rufiji and Morogoro and "rolling out" the products and approaches that led to drastic reductions in mortality in those districts. This challenge is being addressed today, for instance, by a consultancy that has been set up to enable Tanzania's zonal training centres to train and motivate the personnel responsible for bringing those tools and approaches to the rest of Tanzania. "Scaling up," however, is difficult and time-consuming. It is important that we not become discouraged by the scope of this task and that the lessons that flow from the experience in Tanzania — that systemic improvement of health care delivery can greatly reduce mortality — not be discarded or forgotten.

On the web
THE LESSONS

TEHIP Maintains its Momentum

As TEHIP approached the end of its 8-year lifespan, the TEHIP team came to realize that the most difficult work was, in a sense, just beginning.

The discoveries of the past decade all pointed at the new question "what now?" The compelling evidence showing that targeted investments in health systems can dramatically lower mortality would mean little if international agencies and regional and district health planners remained unaware of these findings. And the mechanisms that had been developed to achieve practical gains on the ground — budgeting and planning tools, DSS systems to gather reliable health data, management cascades, etc. — would have minimal impact if they stayed on the shelf and out of the hands of the people responsible for local health planning and delivery. With TEHIP set to fade into history, it became increasingly clear that special efforts were required to ensure that advances made through the "special case" of TEHIP became commonplace features of day-to-day health care delivery over a wider geographic span.

Certainly, the political will to implement meaningful changes to health systems was evident both within Tanzania and beyond its borders. In 2003, delegations from Kenya, Ghana, and Uganda came to Tanzania to observe the progress that had been made in the two test districts and to investigate whether the TEHIP approach could be adapted to their countries. Within Tanzania, meanwhile, health officials were convinced that the TEHIP program should be scaled up nationally. If the results could be replicated outside Rufiji and Morogoro, they calculated, then the health benchmarks set down in the Millennium Development Goals would move within the country's grasp.

Early scaling up

In fact, elements of the TEHIP package had been scaled up well before the end of the project, as a distinct entity, was in sight. Since TEHIP adopted an integrated research and development approach (with the "D" side of the "R&D" amalgam geared to quickly incorporating important research findings into practice) it had been possible to accommodate Ministry of Health (MoH) requests that aspects of a national rollout should proceed before all the long-term project data was in and analyzed. Rigorous scientific evaluation had conclusively demonstrated that certain treatments or interventions were medically safe and effective (although this verification, obviously, was not required before rolling out nonmedical interventions such as the TEHIP tools). Furthermore, TEHIP's preliminary findings had made a convincing case that implementing particular interventions under real-life (and not experimental) conditions could bring down death rates in other districts.

And so — based on information produced in the demonstration districts as early as 1997 — the Ministry had decided to scale up the use of Integrated Management of Childhood Illnesses (IMCI) in 1999, to launch a national campaign promoting the use of insecticide-treated bednets (ITNs) in 2000, and to alter its anti-malarial drug policy (in line with evidence from TEHIP and other data sources) in 2001.

The MoH decision to extend the sector-wide approach (SWAp) budgeting strategy beyond the two test districts was also crucial. This created decentralized District Health Baskets across the country, effectively doubling health spending and enabling districts to apply the appropriate funds to their most pressing health concerns.

The staggered pattern of mortality rate declines in the test districts and in the country as a whole show that moving forward on the rollout of proven interventions, while the TEHIP experiment was still in progress, had been a fruitful decision. While under-5 mortality began dropping in the TEHIP districts in 1998 (eventually reaching a reduction of more than 55% by 2003), statistics reveal falling under-5 deaths nationwide beginning in 2000 (reaching a 40% decline by 2005). The lag of only a few years shows how the Tanzanian government was able to realize broad-based gains by acting, in part, on TEHIP research findings while work in the test districts was still ongoing.

A prototype to inform a national scaling up of TEHIP products was also initiated in advance of TEHIP's closure as a project in mid-2004. In 2003, the United Nations Foundation (UNF) and IDRC funded a 3-year initiative that would move the use of TEHIP tools and strategies beyond the two test districts and into two entire regions — effectively scaling up from 2 to 11 districts. Staff from the Ministry of Health's Zonal Training Centres (ZTCs) were engaged to produce manuals and other materials as the basis for training district health managers in the use of the tools and

On the web
THE LESSONS

front-line health workers in the delivery of new packages of clinical interventions.

This exercise was to be a model for national-level rollout; one of its goals was to identify mechanisms that would aid in the countrywide scale up. It also represented the first time that TEHIP's machinery would be deployed without any involvement by researchers. TEHIP had accomplished its research goals, and it was time to move the resulting products into daily use by health workers in ordinary health facilities across Tanzania — to make those products an integral, functioning part of the country's health infrastructure.

Maintaining momentum

Still, despite this early partial rollout, the approaching closure of TEHIP in 2004 caused some trepidation. There was a realization that concerted and focused action would be required to sustain the momentum that TEHIP had brought to health system revitalization. If TEHIP wound down in the way that development projects typically do — with staff simply packing their bags and moving on to the next challenge — then much of that momentum would surely dissipate. Productive partnerships would be fractured as team members moved on to new jobs and new tasks.

The loss of TEHIP 's budget also posed an obstacle to health officials seeking to institutionalize the lessons of the project, since it was evident that a fresh infusion of resources would be needed to roll out the TEHIP model countrywide, and to train a multitude of health workers who needed to acquire new skills.

There were also fears that TEHIP 's winding-down would trigger a loss of "institutional memory" that would make it more difficult to communicate what had been learned in Rufiji and Morogoro. Researchers might be expected to champion the role of strengthened health systems by publishing papers in scholarly journals, but who would transfer the lessons of TEHIP's years of experimentation to the people responsible for actual service delivery throughout Tanzania, and who would advise officials from elsewhere in Africa seeking to adapt and replicate TEHIP's health gains in their own countries?

Enter the "exit strategy"

Facing these potential setbacks, IDRC and the Tanzanian MoH agreed on a new plan to build on the TEHIP legacy and propel health system renewal further onto the global health agenda. In early 2004, shortly before TEHIP closed its doors, IDRC approved funding for the development of an "exit strategy" that would ensure the orderly transfer of capacities and responsibilities from the project to local institutions, while advancing the training of personnel through the Zonal Training Centre system and encouraging cooperation and coordination among East African states.

Health officials in those states subsequently signaled their support for this policy thrust. In early 2005, the East African Community's Health Ministers endorsed a regional approach linking research evidence with policy development — a statement that led to the ongoing planning for the Regional East African Community Health (REACH) Policy Initiative, designed to strengthen health systems and address cross-border health concerns such as avian flu and Ebola. Then, in mid-2005, Tanzania's Ministry of Health confirmed its commitment to accelerate evidence-based health planning by accepting a plan drawn up by an independent consultancy (funded through the TEHIP Exit Strategy) for strengthening and decentralizing training to enable health workers to participate in TEHIP-style health delivery.

Viewing the full panorama of initiatives arising from the exit strategy, we see a wide span of activities, ranging from the visionary (e.g., planning for the REACH regional health policy initiative and an ambitious revamping of the ZTC system) to the apparently mundane (such as the transfer of TEHIP staff and TEHIP-developed infrastructure to national institutions). Yet each of these components — big and small — made possible the complex task of moving the gains realized in the two-district laboratory of Rufiji and Morogoro beyond those confines and into the wider world.

A well-defined and well-funded exit strategy is a rarity among development projects. It became part of the TEHIP story, however, in response to a realization that the widespread adoption of new methods, tools, and outlooks — even those whose efficacy had been proven convincingly — is not something that would happen by itself. Moving from test case to routine practice would require significant expenditures of time, resources, and thought. Careful planning would be needed to overcome institutional inertia (the reflex to keep doing things the way they have always been done), and to make sure that every part of the system was up to the larger task and that all those components could function together.

IDRC's decision to provide significant funding (approximately CA $2 million) displays an acceptance of the idea that institutionalizing the TEHIP findings would not be an **automatic** process but something that had to be **actively** promoted. This realization was shared by other institutions, such as the Canadian International Development Agency (CIDA), which in November 2005 provided CA $7 million to extend the TEHIP benefits to the rest of the country. Happily, these and other agencies' determination to not simply let the project end (with the risk that its innovations would fall out of use) paid tangible dividends. Building bridges with national, regional, and international institutions appears to have contributed to a new focus on health system strengthening at all those levels. The expansion of evidence-based planning within Tanzania, meanwhile, is moving hand-in-hand with continued improvements in health indicators across the country.

With hindsight, we can categorize the various initiatives undertaken after the TEHIP project closure under the following five thematic banners.

1. Dissemination

TEHIP placed significant emphasis, during its lifespan, on communicating its research findings to practitioners, politicians, communities, donors, and international health authorities through vehicles such as the TEHIP *News* and regular bulletins from the DSS systems. This approach continued during the exit strategy era. PowerPoint presentations, small brochures, newspapers articles — most of them centered on simple, easily understood charts and graphs — were aimed at crucial players in health care reform who likely had neither the time nor the academic background to digest scholarly papers in scientific journals.

After the TEHIP data was in and analyzed, it became essential to ensure that the project's lessons were widely circulated and well understood. Staff focused on communicating clearly expressed health data, as the scaling up proceeded, so that politicians and bureaucrats would become more accustomed to setting policy informed by evidence. They also hoped that this impact on policymakers would move beyond Tanzania — creating a receptive climate across East Africa for implementing evidence-based health care geared to addressing the dominant burdens of disease.

This continued emphasis on dissemination took aim at a problem sometimes referred to as the "know–do gap." In many cases, knowledge of the major causes of illness, of which interventions can most effectively deal with them, and what treatment packages should look like, does exist. Yet there is a chronic gap between this knowledge and what happens in communities. Often, crucial information does not flow to the people who set health policy and deliver health services. Partly, this is a systemic problem stemming from the lack of incentives for translating research findings into usable information that can solve problems: researchers will reap career rewards from publishing papers in scientific journals, but will not benefit from writing short articles that are accessible to health practitioners and policymakers. The "know–do gap" also arises from a discontinuity of roles, wherein no-one is given specific responsibility for ensuring researchers' findings are delivered — in usable form — to the people who design new health policies and deliver health services.

While TEHIP researchers did indeed publish papers in international scientific journals (with the goal of making the case to the global health community that health systems deserve more attention), they also placed special emphasis on communicating TEHIP's findings and recommendations to the often forgotten but important players at the local level. The first edition of *Fixing Health Systems*, published by IDRC in 2004, was also key to reaching policymakers at various levels, as well as agencies and donor partners that would become involved in funding later health system revitalization initiatives.

2. Replication

Since the goal of rolling out new techniques and methods is to strengthen **an existing health system**, scaling up and replicating a project's results is not something that should be undertaken by the project itself, but rather by the health ministry in the host country. In other words, it is important to find existing and appropriate vehicles for delivering innovative health services that are not dependent on the project, but that will survive and flourish after the project has wound down.

The replication of TEHIP's practices and results followed this model. The expanded use of the burden of disease tool and IMCI outside of Rufiji and Morogoro, for example, was instigated by the MoH and accomplished using its institutions. Later, another independent entity (the UNF) joined IDRC in funding the rollout of most of the other interventions to nine additional districts. In doing so, it created the design for a national scale-up process. One key aspect of this exercise was to identify an existing institution within the MoH structure (the Zonal Training Centre system) that could be used — given significant restructuring and revitalization — as the actual machinery for accomplishing a national scale up.

Later in the process — in 2007 — Tanzania's finance ministry incorporated the TEHIP District Health Accounts tool into its PlanRep budgeting software, which all districts are now mandated to use. This is another example of a project tool becoming fully integrated into the national policy-making machinery.

One case where a TEHIP -initiated model is to be replicated outside of Tanzania is the Nigerian Evidence-Based Health System Initiative (NEHSI) — designed by Nigerian and international organizations under the coordination of IDRC, and funded by CIDA and IDRC. Nigeria is the most populated country in sub-Saharan Africa, and one where multiple vertical health programs have created inefficiencies and a lack of coherence in health care delivery. NEHSI will see the creation of DSS systems in two states to compile portraits of the local burden of disease, together with Multi-Stakeholder Information Systems that will ensure ongoing communication among communities, health facilities, planners, researchers, and development partners. This will allow for a more coordinated approach to primary health care planning, delivery, and evaluation, as well as more rational targeting of resources toward the most pressing local health challenges.

3. Planning for sustainability/institutional strengthening

As the sun set on TEHIP, it became essential to transfer knowledge, methods, and capacity — acquired over the project's lifespan — to national, local, and regional institutions. These institutions would be responsible for maintaining the gains that had been achieved during the TEHIP years and for dealing with any new challenges that lay over the horizon.

One entity that took on a large share of that responsibility was the Zonal Training Centre (ZTC) system, which was a virtual institution annexed to an existing health training institution. Like many aspects of the Tanzanian health system, ZTCs were underfunded and in various states of disrepair. The staffing levels were often inadequate, and course content was geared mostly to delivering segregated vertical programs without any coherent, overall vision. Now, the ZTCs are being restructured and reinvigorated through funding allotments from the Ministry and health donor partner basket funds, which includes a CA $7 million grant from CIDA and other individual disbursements from agencies such as the World Bank, DANIDA, GTZ, USAID, JICA, and the Government of the Netherlands.

The importance of the ZTCs to the national scaling up stems from the obvious need to train front-line health workers in new services such as IMCI, which has made a huge contribution to improving children's health outcomes in Tanzania. More broadly, however, the ZTCs offer an entry point in the search for solutions to the recognized and documented crisis in health-sector human resources that plagues most developing countries. Deploying and retaining effective health workers remains one of the most intractable challenges facing the continent's health sector. With low levels of job satisfaction and a lack of incentives (e.g., poor wages and inadequate housing), health workers frequently leave their jobs, relocate to other countries, or take second jobs. Better training through improved ZTCs could represent a first step toward reinstating health workers as valued, respected professionals with a greater stake in their work.

Currently, ZTCs are gearing up for a more streamlined provision of training, wherein practitioners — rather than being pulled out of their workplaces for disconnected training sessions on vertical programs — will learn about key interventions as part of an organized and integrated curriculum. This will also pave the way for a more rational system for allocating and posting health workers in the field. Rather than simply justifying a list for a certain number of health worker cadres, with particular specialized training, it will increasingly be expected that clinical staff will have been trained and have all the required knowledge to deliver the entire national health package on a daily basis.

The ZTCs are also envisioned as a focal point for generating analysis and advice to the ministry. This new role is being defined by the regional centres, which have embarked on a process of creating their own business plans. The enhanced contribution of ZTCs to health management will include activities such as tracking which health workers need retraining or upgrading, providing input to determine what staffing levels are needed in particular areas, and performing follow-up supervision of all trained health workers to ensure high quality performance.

The design and construction of the REACH policy initiative provides another example, at the regional level, of a transfer of knowledge and capacity to a sustainable, ground-level institution. REACH will be the practical expression of the concept that TEHIP staff originally had envisioned as "the Duluti Institute." Its primary function will be to synthesize, package, and distribute health policy options and information to policymakers, so that they are able to undertake more evidence-informed planning and policy-making. Its structure will see individual country nodes (in Tanzania, Kenya, Uganda, Rwanda, and Burundi) linked to a single regional hub at the East African Community level. Requests for information will filter upward from the country levels, so that the regional staff can prepare confidential briefings to inform politicians and bureaucrats on what policy directions the current evidence suggest.

REACH will also deal with cross-border health concerns such as epidemics and the spread of rare or emerging infectious diseases. At the time of this writing, REACH was involved in late-stage fundraising that would allow for a project launch.

Earlier analysis determined that a TEHIP-style approach to health delivery would be best suited to countries where

- there are accessible primary health care facilities within reach of most of the population;

- the health system is to some degree decentralized;

- there is a sector-wide approach (SWAp) funding model in place; and

- some form of health surveillance system exists to provide a foundation for gathering population health data, and there is some national health research capacity.

East African countries such as Uganda, Kenya, and Tanzania (which are participating in REACH) fit that description. Further afield, countries such as Burkina Faso and Zambia also share those characteristics, and thus have the potential to replicate TEHIP-style health delivery.

4. Continued data collection and population health research

The Rufiji DSS station was made financially sustainable and, subsequently, was turned over to the Ifakara Health Research and Development Centre. Another ongoing contribution in the area of data collection has been the establishment, with help from TEHIP, of the INDEPTH network. INDEPTH is comprised of 37 sites operating at the household level in 19 countries in Africa, Asia, Central America, and Oceania. It has produced a "DSS starter kit" to aid in setting up new DSS facilities, works to ensure compatibility of software and operations between different DSS sites, and is encouraging the pooling and comparison of health data across borders.

Gathering reliable health data is an essential cornerstone of evidence-based planning. It not only provides a comprehensive portrait of burden of disease (by capturing all at-home mortality and morbidity as part of the picture), but also provides continual monitoring of health conditions that can rapidly inform whether new types of health delivery or new policies are actually working. This allows health managers to adjust and improve upon the public health package design.

Throughout Africa, the norm for health data collection has been to tally information from cases diagnosed in hospitals and other health facilities, a method that yields incomplete results since many people who are ill stay at home or seek services somewhere else. Partly as a result of TEHIP's example, there is increasing recognition of the crucial contribution of demographic surveillance that incorporates routine population surveys and verbal autopsies for people who have died at home.

This approach is being promoted by a new global health initiative for health information systems — the Health Metrics Network — housed at the WHO. Additionally, the fact that one of NEHSI's main entry points into health system reform in Nigeria is information-gathering through DSS is another demonstration of this new understanding that DSS (or a similar system for gathering population-based health data) is a fundamental requirement for evidence-based health planning in settings where there are no vital events registration systems.

5. Fundraising

With the retirement of TEHIP as an organization, it was important to encourage new donors to step forward and address the multiple needs that had been identified over the course of the project, to build on the project's achievements, and to address new stresses and bottlenecks that the health system will inevitably suffer.

New infusions of funds and expressions of commitment have indeed improved the prospects for health system renewal in sub-Saharan Africa. For example, Comic Relief, a UK charity whose previous concern had been largely with providing relief after events such as natural disasters, has ventured into the more complex matter of health system strengthening by awarding the Ifakara Centre a (UK) £5 million grant over 5 years. (This was the largest grant ever awarded by Comic Relief, and it makes Ifakara the first African institution that Comic Relief has funded directly.) With input from the original TEHIP team, Ifakara submitted a proposal to Comic Relief for a project seeking to replicate the kind of gains made by TEHIP in under-5 child health, by using the R&D approach to obtain similar improvements in maternal and neonatal care, both areas where the death rate remains unacceptably high. From the outset, Comic Relief had expressed a desire to back project designs that incorporated TEHIP methods, particularly the integration of research and development in actual field conditions.

In addition to linking research directly to development, this Comic Relief-funded work has many other characteristics that were hallmarks of TEHIP. It will address recognized needs and priorities set out by the Ministry of Health, and will engage researchers in partnership with district planners, front-line health staff, and communities. It will use DSS resources to monitor ongoing progress and will attempt to review and update existing TEHIP planning tools. It is not bound by short-term time restrictions and targets, but will allow for the pace of work to be dictated by conditions on the ground. It will feed results back to the Zonal Training Centres, so that advances in maternal and neonatal health will be incorporated into training and will inform policy and practice across the nation.

There are several other examples of organizations picking up where TEHIP left off — taking the growing interest in the links between improved health systems and better health to new frontiers, both geographically and conceptually. For example:

- The US-based Doris Duke Foundation is providing US $100 million in grants for health system research and development in Ghana, Kenya, Lesotho, Madagascar, Malawi, Mozambique, Rwanda, Tanzania, and Zambia.

- CIDA has launched a CA $450 million "African Health Systems Initiative" to help strengthen health systems across sub-Saharan Africa.

- The Wellcome Trust (UK) has joined with IDRC and the UK's Department for International Development to provide support for health research capacity strengthening, including initiatives specifically focused on linking research to health policy, to strengthen health systems in Malawi and Kenya. Each country is due to receive approximately £11 million from the donor consortium over 5 years.

Those examples reflect a growing consensus that operational questions need to be addressed if Africa is to make significant strides toward achieving the MDGs. While 10 years ago, most health investment flowed to the development of new vaccines or other technological fixes, there is a growing focus on answering systemic questions such as how to remove the barriers that prevent health care from reaching the people who need it; how health packages can be better designed and delivered; and how improved personnel, transportation, and related logistical practices can help health systems do what they were intended to do.

These sorts of questions are now being asked at the highest levels. In 2004, for example, the WHO's *World Report on Knowledge for Better Health* called for more innovative health system research to help bridge "the know-do gap." In short, the world has changed since TEHIP set out to test the 1993 *World Development Report* hypothesis that modest investments in health systems could produce significant improvements in health.

Still, this new and promising climate does not justify complacency. Having mechanisms in place to improve health care delivery does not mean there will not be new challenges and setbacks. The factors that affect population health are dynamic and ever-changing. Managing health systems to respond to shifting needs and variations in the relative burdens of disease requires continuous attention to a large number of factors, but even still, unexpected circumstances may arise that can derail even the most carefully laid plans.

It is also likely that a particular package of interventions, after producing dramatic results, may hit a "plateau" where improvements in health outcomes start to level out. This has been the story in Tanzania, where DSS data are suggesting that most of the improvements that can be expected from IMCI have already occurred. When the health system hits this kind of "hard floor " — when the illness and death rates in a particular category seem to have become intransigent or fixed — this is the time when health planners must look to other areas where mortality levels can be brought down to similar levels. In other words, when the low-hanging fruit has been picked off the tree, it's time to buy a ladder and start picking higher up.

This is what is happening in Tanzania, where health planners are now looking to improve outcomes in neonatal and maternal health. While under-5 deaths began to decline steeply in 1999, neonatal and maternal death rates remained constant (Figure 7). For further declines in under-5 mortality — needed to achieve the Millennium Development Goals — it is clear that greater efforts are needed on both neonatal mortality and maternal mortality. Making gains in these areas will be essential if Tanzania is to make the necessary strides toward achieving the MDGs related to child and maternal health.

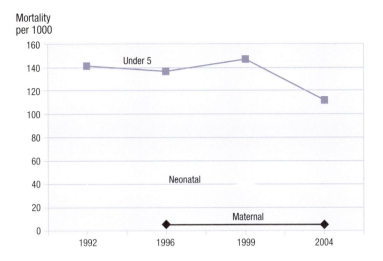

Figure 7. **Under-5, neonatal, and maternal mortality in Tanzania, 1992–2004.**

In short, there are no "quick fixes" or "silver bullets" in the quest to reduce Africa's unacceptably high death rates. Having an effective, functioning health system in place is merely one crucial stage in an ongoing process that requires continual vigilance, attention to a large range of details, and a willingness to tackle the new challenges. Having the proper tools at the ready will provide health planners with the means to improve population health. But making sure those tools are used to greatest effect will also require ingenuity, commitment, and sustained political will.

Acknowledgments

A project of this magnitude and timescale benefits from the contributions of an enormous number of people. First, we would like to draw attention to some of TEHIP's key supporters and contributors. This is followed by a more complete list of contributors.

Members of the International Advisory Committee, chaired by Dr Joe Cook, provided direction and support during the initial EHIP design phase. We wish to particularly highlight our appreciation for the significant conceptual contributions made by the late Jose Luis Bobadilla of the World Bank. Valuable design inputs were also provided by members of the Scientific Advisory Committee under the Chairmanship of Dr Demissie Habte. We are indebted to the former EHIP executive directors Joel Finlay and Irene Mathias and for IDRC liaison through Drs Eva Rathgeber, Connie Freeman, and Christina Zarowsky and to former EHIP staff, most notably Karen Madden and Kaye Meikle.

At the Tanzanian Ministry of Health, TEHIP has benefited from the unflagging support of the Honourable Minister Anna M. Abdullah, the former Ministers Dr Aaron Chiduo and Ms Zakia Meghji, Permanent Secretary Ms M.J. Mwaffisi, Chief Medical Officer Dr G.L. Upunda, and Ministry of Health Directors Dr G. Mliga, Mr E.N. Manumbu, and Dr Ali A. Mzige. We are grateful for the contributions of Dr Peter Kilima, former Director of Preventive Services and District Medical Officers, Dr Harun Machibya and Dr Saidi Mkikima, and their District Health Management Teams. Rufiji District Executive Director Mr F.Q.M. Fissoo and Morogoro District Executive Director John Gille have been key partners. Extending TEHIP's gains to the rest of the country is a task in the able hands of Ministry staff from the zonal training centres, notably Drs S.R. Fundikira, S. Ndeki, C. Jincen, and B.Y. Ndawi.

Funding was provided by Canada's International Development Research Centre (IDRC), the Canadian International Development Agency (CIDA), the World Bank, and the Ministry of Health of Tanzania. The Tanzanian Ministry of Health is currently undertaking a regional roll-out of TEHIP tools with funding contributed by the United Nations Foundation and administered by the World Health Organization (WHO). TEHIP would not have been possible without the vision and efforts of the former IDRC Director of Health Sciences, Dr Maureen Law. Thank you to TEHIP's administrative and financial team, under the direction of Mr Godfrey Munna. We also gratefully acknowledge assistance from the Canadian High Commission, the CIDA office in Dar es Salaam, and the WHO Tanzania office, particularly former WHO country representatives Dr Dirk Warning and Dr Wedson Mwambazi and current representative Dr Edward Maganu.

TEHIP's successes have relied on the specific expertise of many people. Among them are Dr M.V. Meshack and his team at the University College of Land and Architectural Studies, who contributed to the community rehabilitation tool. Mr Jacques Wilmo of CT/BA Ltd provided excellent software design for cost tracking. WHO contributed technical support for the Integrated Management of Childhood Illnesses program through Dr Leslie Mgalula and the Iringa Primary Health Care Institute was responsible for adapting WHO's manual for strengthening health management in districts and provinces. We thank Dr Andrew Kitua, Director General of the National Institute for Medical Research, and his predecessor, Prof. Wen Kilama, for permission to conduct the research.

TEHIP's National Steering Committee drew its members from the Government of Tanzania, IDRC, WHO, UNICEF, the World Bank, and CIDA. Tanzanian technical partners include the Ifakara Health Research Development Centre under the leadership of Dr Hassan Mshinda, the Muhimbili College of Health Sciences, the Institute of Public Health through the late Dr George Lwihula, and the University of Dar es Salaam's Institute of Development Studies through Dr Peter Kamuzora. Mr William Lobulu, assisted by Mr Sydney Kwiyamba, provided excellent editorial work for TEHIP communications. IDRC's Communications Division facilitated the creation and production of this book and the associated Web portal: **http://www.idrc.ca/tehip**.

Finally, we also thank the people and health workers of Rufiji and Morogoro, who contributed greatly to the rebuilding of their districts' health care systems and who now benefit from the ongoing health care reforms.

It is impossible to acknowledge every single contributor to TEHIP's achievements but we particularly want to highlight both the individuals and teams set out below.

Conceptual design

The overall conceptual design of EHIP was put in place by its initial **Steering Committee**: Jose Luis Bobadilla, World Bank; Joe Cook, Edna McConnell Clark Foundation; Don de Savigny,

IDRC; Joel Finlay, IDRC; Tore Godal, WHO; Demissie Habte, International Centre for Diarrhoeal Disease Research, Bangladesh; Dean Jamison, World Bank; Michel Jancloes, WHO; Steve Jarrett, UNICEF; Maureen Law, IDRC; Ernest Loevinsohn, CIDA; Tom Nchinda, WHO; Ebrahim Samba, WHO; Rogatian Shirima, Ministry of Health, Tanzania; Jim Tulloch, WHO.

As EHIP took root in Tanzania, the International Steering Committee evolved to an **International Advisory Committee**: Agnes Aidoo, UNICEF; Joe Cook, Edna-McConnell Clark Foundation; Joel Finlay, IDRC; Charles Griffen, World Bank; Maureen Law, IDRC; Irene Mathias, IDRC; Don McMaster, CIDA; Raymond Mrope, Ministry of Health, Tanzania; Eva Rathgeber, IDRC; Ebrahim Samba, WHO; Jim Tulloch, WHO; Dirk Warning, WHO.

Once work commenced on the ground in Tanzania, the International Advisory Committee evolved to a **National Steering Committee**: Adeline Kimambo, Ministry of Health, Tanzania; Emmanual Malangalila, World Bank, Tanzania; R. Mariki, Tanzania Planning Commission; Ben Moses, Prime Minister's Office, Tanzania; Raymond Mrope, Ministry of Health, Tanzania; Victoria Mushi, CIDA Tanzania; S. Sijaona, Prime Minister's Office, Tanzania; Gabriel Upunda, Ministry of Health, Tanzania; Dirk Warning, WHO Tanzania.

Research design

Although research and development are inextricably linked, much effort was invested in developing a research design that would hold plausibility for policymakers and planners. The conceptualization of TEHIP research emerged from a series of consultative workshops held in Ottawa in July 1994, Geneva in October 1994, Washington in February 1995, and Morogoro in July 1995 attended variously by Neil Andersson, CIET International; Elizabeth Badley, University of Toronto; Essy Banniasad, Dalhousie University; Enis Baris, IDRC; Fred Binka, Ministry of Health, Ghana;

Robert Black, John Hopkins University; Jose Luis Bobadilla, World Bank; Mariam Claeson, WHO; Peter Cowley, World Bank; Don de Savigny, IDRC; Timothy Evans, Harvard University; Joel Finlay, IDRC; Pierre Fournier, University of Montreal; Larry Gelmon, IDRC; Lucy Gilson, London School of Hygiene and Tropical Medicine; Tore Godal, WHO; Demissie Habte, International Centre for Diarrhoeal Disease Research, Bangladesh; Margaret Hillson, Canadian Public Health Association; Dean Jamison, World Bank; Harun Kasale, TEHIP; Peter Kilima, Ministry of Health, Tanzania; Henry Kitange, Ministry of Health, Tanzania; Maureen Law, IDRC; Nicolaus Lorenz, Swiss Tropical Institute; Wilbald Lorri, Tanzania Food and Nutrition Centre; Karen Madden, IDRC; Conrad Mbuya, TEHIP; Anne Mills, London School of Hygiene and Tropical Medicine; Bertha Mo, IDRC; Lawrence Munyetti, Ministry of Health, Tanzania; Christopher Murray, Harvard University; Marguerite Pappaioanou, US Centres for Disease Control; Dev Ray, WHO; Peter Riwa, Ministry of Health, Tanzania; David Ross, London School of Hygiene and Tropical Medicine; Joas Rugemalila, Tanzania National Institute of Medical Research; Steve Sapire, WHO; Sally Stansfield, McGill University; George Stroh, US Centres for Disease Control; Marcel Tanner, Swiss Tropical Institute; Peter Tugwell, University of Ottawa; Gerome van Ginneken, Netherlands Interdisciplinary Demographic Unit; Gabriel Upunda, Ministry of Health, Tanzania; Cesar Victora, Federal University of Pelotas; Russell Wilkins, Health Canada; Dennis Willms, McMaster University.

The general scope and core protocols for component A (health systems) and component B (health behaviours) were prepared by an ad hoc group convened in Basel in May 1996 by a subcommittee of the Scientific Advisory Committee. The group consisted of Doug Angus, University of Ottawa; Fred Binka, Ministry of Health, Ghana; Don de Savigny, IDRC; David Evans, WHO; Lucy Gilson, University of Witswatersrand; Andrew Kitua, Ifakara Health Research and Development Centre; George Lwihula, Muhimbili Medical Centre; Conrad Mbuya, TEHIP; Graham Reid,

IDRC; Marcel Tanner, Swiss Tropical Institute; Mitchell Weiss, Swiss Tropical Institute; Dennis Willms, McMaster University.

The approach to component C (demographic surveillance) emerged from a workshop on DSS methods held in Dar es Salaam in February 1996 attended by Joanna Armstrong-Schellenberg, Ifakara Health Research and Development Centre; Sandra Baldwin, UK Office for Development Assistance (now the UK Department for International Development); Fred Binka, Ministry of Health, Ghana; Don de Savigny, IDRC; Andrew Hall, Oxford University; Harun Kasale, TEHIP; Peter Kilima, Ministry of Health, Tanzania; Japhet Killewo, Muhimbili College of Health Sciences; John Kimario, Ifakara Health Research and Development Centre; Henry Kitange, Adult Morbidity and Mortality Project (AMMP), Ministry of Health, Tanzania; Zohra Lukmanji, Tanzania Food and Nutrition Centre; Harun Machibya, Ministry of Health, Tanzania; Cheick Mbacke, Rockefeller Foundation; Conrad Mbuya, TEHIP; Bruce McLeod, University of Maryland; Leslie Mgalula, WHO/TEHIP; Candida Moshiro, Muhimbili Medical Centre; Sadiki Mshana, Ministry of Health, Tanzania; Robert Mswia, AMMP, Ministry of Health, Tanzania; Lawrence Munyetti, Ministry of Health, Tanzania; Rose Nathan, Ifakara Health Research and Development Centre; Chris Nevill, African Medical and Research Foundation; Sylvester Ngalaba, Tanzania Bureau of Statistics; Pierre Ngom, Ministry of Health, Navrongo, Ghana; Jim Phillips, Population Council; David Ross, London School of Hygiene and Tropical Medicine; Daudi Simba, Ministry of Health, Tanzania; Michael Strong, Ethiopia National Office of Population; Nigel Unwin, University of Newcastle; David Whiting, AMMP, Ministry of Health, Tanzania; Susan Zimicki, Harvard Institute for International Development.

Overall guidance to the execution of TEHIP research has been provided since April 1996 by a **Scientific Advisory Committee**: Jose Luis Bobadilla, World Bank; Peter Cowley, US Agency for International Development; Don de Savigny, IDRC; David Evans,

WHO; Sandy Gove, WHO; Demissie Habte, World Bank (Chair); Sylvia Kaaya, Muhimbili University College of Health Sciences; Andrew Kitua, National Institute for Medical Research; Wilbald Lorri, Tanzania Food and Nutrition Centre; Conrad Mbuya, TEHIP; Winnie Mpanju-Shumbusho, Commonwealth Regional Health Community; Fatma Mrisho, United Nations Population Fund; Gernard Msamanga, Muhimbili University College of Health Sciences; Lawrence Munyetti, Ministry of Health, Tanzania; Raphael Owor, Makerere University; Eva Rathgeber, IDRC; David Ross, London School of Hygiene and Tropical Medicine; Daniel Sala-Diakanda, United Nations Economic Commission for Africa; Marcel Tanner, Swiss Tropical Institute; Cesar Victora, Federal University of Pelotas; Dennis Willms, McMaster University.

TEHIP-supported researchers

Health systems research: Dr Peter Kamuzora, Institute of Development Studies, University of Dar es Salaam; Mr Phares Mujinja, Institute of Public Health, Muhimbli University College of Health Sciences; Mr Cyprian Makwaya, Institute of Public Health, Muhimbli University College of Health Sciences; Dr Innocent Semali, Institute of Public Health, University College of Health Sciences.

Health behaviour research: Dr George Lwihula, Institute of Public Health, Muhimbili University College of Health Sciences; Mr Charles Mayombana, Ifakara Health Research and Development Centre; Mr Ahmed Makemba, Ifakara Health Research and Development Centre; Dr Felician Tungaraza, Department of Sociology, University of Dar es Salaam; Ms Joyce Nyoni, Department of Sociology, University of Dar es Salaam.

Health impact research: Dr Eleuther Mwageni, Station Manager, Rufiji DSS, Ikwiriri; Mr Zaharani Juma, Data Manager, Rufiji DSS, Ikwiriri; Mr Mohamed Irema, Field Manager, Rufiji DSS, Ikwiriri; the TEHIP and AMMP teams

A final word of thanks to the dedicated TEHIP office and support staff, who have included, since 1996, Godfrey Munna, Robert Kilala, Steria Cosmas, Elimamba Tenga, Frida Zimamoto, the late Victor Lihendeko, Herieth Julius, Rose Lusinde, Faustina Daniel, Mohammed Njechele, Jamal Mkunguru, Bakari Ali, the late Alice Mmari, and Gladys Githaiga.

Glossary of Terms and Acronyms

AFI: Acute febrile illness

Alma-Ata Conference: Alma-Ata International Conference on Primary Health Care, held 6–12 September 1978, in Alma-Ata, USSR. The first such international conference, it was sponsored by the World Health Organization and UNICEF and attended by delegates from 134 countries. It presented the manifesto to attain global health for the 21st century by providing basic health care aimed at the urban and rural poor of the developing world.

AMMP: Adult Morbidity and Mortality Project. A joint project of the Tanzania Ministry of Health and the University of Newcastle Upon Tyne, funded by the Department for International Development, United Kingdom.

BCG: Bacillus of Calmette-Guérin vaccine, administered by injection to protect against tuberculosis.

Burden of Disease Profile: An annual document used in planning and priority setting that graphically presents population health information from a sentinel Demographic Surveillance System in easily understood computer-generated charts and tables. It presents results not in terms of individual diseases, but in terms of aggregated intervention-addressable shares of the burden of disease.

Child survival revolution: An initiative launched by James Grant, Executive Director of UNICEF, in its December 1982 *State of the World's Children* report. The initiative later included child development. Through this initiative, UNICEF proposed to vanquish common infections of early childhood using simple, low-cost technologies: growth monitoring, oral rehydration therapy for diarrhoea, breastfeeding, and immunization against the 6 vaccine-preventable childhood killers: tuberculosis, diphtheria, whooping cough, tetanus, polio, and measles.

CIDA: Canadian International Development Agency

Community voice tool: An approach known as participatory action research that can assist in bringing the demands of the community into the district planning process.

Cost-effectiveness: The cost to avert the loss of a Disability Adjusted Life Year.

DALY: Disability Adjusted Life Years. The DALY extends the concept of potential years of life lost due to premature death to include years of "healthy" life lost by virtue of being in states of ill-health. DALYs for a disease or risk factor are calculated as the annual sum of the years of life lost due to premature mortality in the population and the "years lived with disability" for incident cases of the health condition.

DANIDA: Danish International Development Agency

Declaration of Alma-Ata: A manifesto issued at the close of the September 1978 Alma-Ata Conference on Primary Health Care, which stated that "This conference strongly reaffirms that health is a state of complete physical, mental and social well being and not merely the absence of disease or infirmity ... A major social target of governments, international organizations and the whole world community in the coming decades should be the attainment by all people of the world by the year 2000 of a level of health that will permit them to lead socially and economically productive lives."

DHMT: District Health Management Team. A key component of Tanzania's health sector reforms was the establishment of DHMTs in each of the country's 123 districts. Comprised of members with complementary skills and multiple areas of expertise, DMHTs are responsible for health planning, managing, and monitoring. (Now called Council Health Management Teams in Tanzania.)

District Cost Information System: A custom database managed at the district level and used to store information from the Health Management Information System (HMIS), including the sex, age group, in/out patient status, repeat patient status, and diagnosis, as well as the drugs, surgical procedures, and laboratory tests prescribed. Its primary purpose is to identify technical efficiency in the delivery of essential clinical and public health interventions.

District Health Accounts Tool, also known as the District Health Expenditures Mapping Tool: A customized Microsoft Excel application designed to help DHMTs analyze their budgets and expenditures by providing a one-page analytical summary and several graphical "pictures" of key aspects of their annual plan.

District Health Service Mapping Tool: A simplified "point and click" geographic information (GIS) software application designed by WHO. Called HealthMapper, it is used to facilitate entry of HMIS data into a district level database and its graphical display on local maps of the district.

DOTS: Directly Observed Treatment — Short Course.

DSS: Demographic Surveillance System. A method of continuously monitoring a geographically defined population to provide timely data on all births, deaths, causes of deaths, and migrations.

EDP: Essential Drugs Program

EHIP: Essential Health Interventions Project, precursor of TEHIP.

EPI: Expanded Program on Immunization

Global Fund to Fight AIDS, Tuberculosis and Malaria: A fund established in January 2002 to dramatically increase resources to fight three of the world's most devastating diseases, and to direct those resources to areas of greatest need. An outgrowth of work undertaken by the G-8 group of countries, leaders of African states, and UN Secretary General Kofi Annan, it is a partnership between governments, civil society, the private sector, and affected communities.

G-8: Group of 8. An informal group of 8 countries — Canada, France, Germany, Italy, Japan, Russia, the United Kingdom, and the United States. Each year, G-8 leaders and representatives from the European Union meet to discuss broad economic and foreign policies.

HealthMapper: See District Health Service Mapping Tool.

HMIS: Health Management Information System. A system to collect routine data from hospitals and community health facilities.

HIV/AIDS: Human Immunodeficiency Virus/Acquired Immune Deficiency Syndrome

IDRC: International Development Research Centre, Canada

IEC: Information, education, and communication

IMAI: Integrated Management of Adolescent and Adult Illness. A health care strategy that focuses on the main clinical conditions that account for most adolescent and adult deaths and disability across the world, and integrates the prevention of illness and care of the adolescent and adult in a single health care package. This includes pneumonia, malaria, sexually transmitted infections, key women's health issues, mental health disorders, and the detection and care of priority chronic conditions that can be prevented or treated with cost-effective measures, such as epilepsy, tuberculosis, and HIV.

IMC: Integrated Management Cascade. A hierarchical communications and supervisory structure that allows delegation of responsibilities from the DHMT level down to the lower levels of the district health system.

IMCI: Integrated Management of Childhood Illnesses: A health strategy developed by WHO and UNICEF that targets children under 5 and addresses 5 leading causes of death — malaria, pneumonia, diarrhoea, measles, and malnutrition.

INDEPTH Network: An international network of field sites with continuous demographic evaluation of populations and their health. This umbrella organization embraces 40 field sites in Africa, Southeast Asia, and Oceania. Their focus includes data analysis and capacity strengthening, technical support to field sites, comparative assessments of mortality, and equity with and emphasis on applications to policy and practice.

Intervention-addressable shares of burden of disease: A method of expressing burden of disease data in terms of the aggregated percentage of disease burden addressed by available, cost-effective interventions (for example, IMCI would address the combined burden of disease in children under 5 years of age caused by malaria, pneumonia, diarrhoea, malnutrition, and measles).

ITNs: Insecticide-treated mosquito netting.

MDGs: United Nations Millennium Development Goals. A set of 8 goals adopted in September 2000 that bind countries to do more and join forces in the fight against poverty, illiteracy, hunger, lack of education, gender inequality, child and maternal mortality, disease, and environmental degradation. The goals set targets to be achieved by 2015.

MoH: Ministry of Health

NEHSI: Nigerian Evidence-Based Health Systems Initiative

NGO: Nongovernmental organization

PAR: Participatory action research

Plausibility design: A rigorous method of summative evaluation of health interventions or programs, as delivered in real-life health systems, that assesses the program's utilization, coverage, or impact. The objective is to provide plausible inferences to decision-makers and policymakers. The approach may use historical, internal or external control groups and places a heavy emphasis on contextual factors. It answers the question: did the program have an effect above and beyond what may have been caused by other external factors?

Population health: The health, well-being, and functioning of a clearly defined population. "The health outcomes of a group of individuals, including the distribution of such outcomes within the groups" (Kindig and Stoddart 2003).

REACH: Regional East African Community Health

Roll Back Malaria Partnership: A global initiative — made up of more than 90 partners — whose goal is to halve the burden of malaria by 2010. The partnership was launched in 1998 by the World Health Organization, UNICEF, UNDP, and the World Bank to provide a coordinated international approach to fighting malaria.

SAPs: Structural adjustment programs. Created in the late 1970s, SAPs are aimed at changing the structure of a developing country's economy to correct underlying problems that lead to economic declines. Initiated by the World Bank, structural adjustment programs aim to increase developing countries' ability to service their international debt and have generally increased privatization of government functions and increased support for export production of agriculture commodities.

SMI: Safe Motherhood Initiative

STD: Sexually transmitted disease

SWAp: Sector-wide approach. A SWAp is a process in which funding for the sector — from both government and donor partner — is conducted in partnership as a means to increase donor-government collaboration, consolidate local management of resources, and undertake the policy and systems reform necessary to achieve a greater impact on health issues.

TEHIP: Tanzania Essential Health Interventions Project

TZS: Tanzanian shilling (in 2004, 1 USD = 1 094 TZS)

UNAIDS: Joint United Nations Programme on HIV/AIDS

UNESCO: United Nations Educational, Scientific and Cultural Organization

UNF: United Nations Foundation

UNICEF: United Nations Children's Fund

Verbal autopsy: A method of assigning the cause of death based on an interview with next of kin or other caregivers.

Village health account: An account established by villages to fund health-related activities and to which villagers contribute through local taxes on their products.

WDR93: *World Development Report 1993: Investing in Health*, published by the World Bank.

WHO: World Health Organization

YLLs: Years of life lost. A measure of time lost due to premature death.

ZTC: Zonal Training Centre (also known as Zonal Continuing Education Centre) A number of institutions set up and run by the Ministry of Health distributed across the country, to provide continuing health education to the various levels of health managers and health personnel.

Sources and Resources

The focus of this book is the Tanzanian Essential Health Interventions Project (TEHIP), a collaboration of IDRC and the Tanzanian Ministry of Health that has helped guide the reform of the health sector in Tanzania and has led to new tools and strategies for maximizing the health benefits of investing in health care. This book does not intend to provide a review of all the pertinent literature and resources for this subject, however this appendix offers a small selection of resources for further background information.

This book is also an integral part of IDRC's thematic Web dossier on the TEHIP experience: **http://www.idrc.ca/tehip**. The full text of the book is available online and leads the reader to other resources on the experience of TEHIP and its partners and collaborators, the tools and strategies arising from the program, and the larger health care issues facing sub-Saharan Africa. Those additional resources include a series of short videos, case studies, and a wide selection of documents. A number of more formal peer-reviewed publications are in the pipeline as of the publication date of this book. Links to these will be available on the Web site as they become available.

Cited references

Bobadilla, J.L.; Cowley, P.; Musgrove, P.; Saxenian, H. 1994. Design, content and financing of an essential national package of health services. Bulletin of the World Health Organization, 72, 653–662. **http://whqlibdoc.who.int/bulletin/1994/Vol72-No4/bulletin_1994_72(4)_653-662.pdf**

Cassels, A.; Janovsky, K. 1995. Strengthening health management in districts and provinces. World Health Organization, Geneva, Switzerland. pp. 1–73.

Commission on Macroeconomics and Health. 2001. Macroeconomics and health: investing in health for economic development. World Health Organization, Geneva, Switzerland. **http://www.cid.harvard.edu/cidcmh/CMHReport.pdf**

Conference Board of Canada. 2004. Understanding health care cost drivers and escalators. Conference Board of Canada, Ottawa, Canada.

de Savigny, D.; Mayombana, C.; Mwageni, E.; Masanja, H.; Minhaj, A.; Mkilindi, Y.; Mbuya, C.; Kasale, H.; Reid, G. 2004. Care-seeking patterns for fatal malaria in Tanzania. Malaria Journal, 3, 27. **http://www.malariajournal.com/content/3/1/27**

Iringa Primary Health Care Institute. 1997. Ten steps to a district health plan: a workbook for district health management teams (revised edition). Iringa Primary Health Care Institute, Iringa, Tanzania / Nijmegen Institute for International Health, University of Nijmegen, Nijmegen, Netherlands.

Kindig, D.A.; Stoddart, G. 2003. What is population health? American Journal of Public Health, 93, 380–383.

Kurowski, C.; Wyss, K.; Abdulla, S.; Yémadji, N.; Mills, A. 2003. Human resources for health: requirements and availability in the context of scaling-up priority interventions in low-income countries – case studies from Tanzania and Chad. London School of Hygiene and Tropical Medicine, London, UK. HEFP working paper 01/04.

Lengeler, C.; Cattani, J.; de Savigny, D. 1996. Net gain: a new method for preventing malaria deaths. International Development Research Centre, Ottawa, Canada. **http://web.idrc.ca/en/ ev-9338-201-1-DO_TOPIC.html**

TEHIP (Tanzania Essential Health Interventions Project). 1998. TEHIP research: scope and approaches. TEHIP, International Development Research Centre, Ottawa, Canada. **http://network.idrc.ca/en/ev-62098-201-1-DO_TOPIC.html**

UNICEF (United Nations Children's Fund). 1996. The state of the world's children. UNICEF, New York, NY, USA. **http://www.unicef.org/sowc96/1980s.htm**

World Bank. 1993. World development report 1993: investing in health. World Bank, Washington, DC, USA.

WHO (World Health Organization). 2000. The World Health Report 2000. Health systems: improving performance. WHO, Geneva, Switzerland. pp. 1–206. **http://www.who.int/ whr2001/2001/archives/200/en/index.html**

WHO (World Health Organization) and UNICEF (United Nations Children's Fund). 1978. Declaration of Alma-Ata. International Conference on Primary Health Care, Alma-Ata, USSR, 6–12 September 1978. WHO, Geneva, Switzerland. http://www.who.int/hpr/NPH/docs/declaration_almaata.pdf

___ 2004. World report on knowledge for better health: strengthening health systems. WHO, Geneva, Switzerland.

Selected Web sites

The following organizations and initiatives are involved with health research and health systems development in Africa:

World Health Organization: **http://www.who.int**

Health, Nutrition and Population (World Bank): **http://www1.worldbank.org/hnp**

The Alliance for Health Policy and Systems Research: **http://www.alliance-hpsr.org/jahia/Jahia**

The Alliance's search engine for health and policy systems research is an excellent source of African health information: **http://white.collexis.net/collexis_evidencebase/www**

Commission on Macroeconomics and Health (WHO): **http://www.who.int/macrohealth**

The Global Fund to Fight AIDS, Tuberculosis and Malaria: **http://www.theglobalfund.org**

Roll Back Malaria (WHO): **http://www.rbm.who.int**

Bill and Melinda Gates Foundation: **http://www.gatesfoundation.org**

Rockefeller Foundation: **http://www.rockfound.org**

The Wellcome Trust: **http://www.wellcome.ac.uk**

United Nations Foundation: **http://www.unfoundation.org**

Council for Health Research for Development: **http://www.cohred.ch**

Global Forum for Health Research: **http://www.globalforumhealth.org**

Governance, Equity, and Health (IDRC): **http://www.idrc.ca/geh**

Demographic and Health Surveys: **http://www.measuredhs.com**

INDEPTH (International Network of field sites with continuous Demographic Evaluation of Populations and Their Health in developing countries): **http://www.indepth-network.org**

International Clinical Epidemiology Network: **http://www.inclen.org**

Further reading

Comprehensive identification and access to published materials dealing with many topics discussed in this book can be found by using the search engine available at **http://www.ncbi.nlm.nih.gov/PubMed**.

More information on the UN Millennium Development Goals (MDGs) is available at **http://www.un.org/millenniumgoals**. Information on MDGs as related to Tanzania is available in the Tanzania country report: **http://www.undg.org/documents/2745-International_Millennium.pdf**.

Parallel preparatory World Bank, WHO, and other documents appearing at the same time as WDR93 and of great influence, specifically for Africa, were the following:

World Bank. 1994. Better health in Africa: experience and lessons learned. World Bank, Washington, DC, USA. Development in Practice series.

Feachem, R.; Jamison, D.T., ed. 1991. Disease and mortality in sub-Saharan Africa. Oxford University Press, Oxford, UK.

Jamison, D.T., et al., ed. 1993. Disease control priorities in developing countries. Oxford Medical Publications, Oxford, UK.

Murray, C.J.L.; Lopez. A.D. 1994. Global comparative assessments in the health sector: disease burden, expenditures and intervention packages. World Health Organization, Geneva, Switzerland.

For information pertaining to the startup of TEHIP:

Finlay, J.; Law, M.; Gelmon, L; de Savigny, D. 1995. A new Canadian health care initiative in Tanzania. Canadian Medical Association Journal, 153, 1081–1085. An abstract of this article can be found at **http://www.cmaj.ca/cgi/content/ abstract/153/8/1081**.

IDRC; World Bank; WHO. 1993. Future partnership for the acceleration of health development: report of a conference, 18–20 October 1993, Ottawa, Canada. IDRC, Ottawa, Canada. **http://web.idrc.ca/en/ev-64424-201-1-DO_TOPIC.html**

For contemporary statistical information on Tanzania:

The official Government of Tanzania Web site, **http://www.tanzania.go.tz**, for links to statistical databases including the 2002 census and the household budget survey

The Muhimbili Health Exchange Forum: **http://www.muhef.or.tz**

The Adult Morbidity and Mortality Project: **http://www.ncl.ac.uk/ammp**

The Tanzania Development Gateway:
http://www.developmentgateway.org/node/285491/

A wealth of information on the international applications of
Demographic Surveillance Systems can be found at
http://www.indepth-network.net. For more information:

INDEPTH Network. 2002. Population and health in developing
countries. Volume 1: Population, health, and survival at
INDEPTH sites. IDRC, Ottawa, Canada.
http://web.idrc.ca/en/ev-9435-201-1-DO_TOPIC.html

Pepall, J. 2002. Vital statistics. IDRC Reports, Ottawa, Canada.
http://web.idrc.ca/en/ev-26044-201-1-DO_TOPIC.html

Mwageni, E.; Masanja, H.; Juma, Z.; Momburi, D.; Mkilindi,
Y.; Mbuya, C.; Kasale, H.; Reid, G.; de Savigny, D. 2004. Socioeconomic status and health inequalities in rural Tanzania: evidence from the Rufiji Demographic Surveillance System.
INDEPTH Network, Accra, Ghana. In press.

More information on the Integrated Management of Childhood
Illnesses (IMCI) can be found at **http://www.who.int/child-
adolescent-health/integr.htm** and at **http://www.who.int/
imci-mce**.

More information on malaria interventions is available at the
Roll Back Malaria Web site: **http://www.rbm.who.int**.

Articles on the management and planning tools developed by
TEHIP and offered to district health teams can be found in various
issues of *TEHIP News*: **http://web.idrc.ca/en/ev-8331-201-1-
DO_TOPIC.html**.

For more information related to the tools and priority setting:

de Savigny, D.; Kasale, H.; Mbuya, C.; Lusinde, R.; Munna, G.;
Masanja, H.; Mgalula, L.; Reid, G. 2003. Choosing health
interventions and setting priorities: a district level perspective.

Medicus Mundi Schweiz. Netzwerk Gesundheit fur alle. Bulletin, 91, 25–30.

de Savigny, D.; Wijeyaratne, P., ed. 1995. GIS for health and the environment. IDRC, Ottawa, Canada. **http://web.idrc.ca/en/ev-9357-201-1-DO_TOPIC.html**

For general information on TEHIP and the various aspects of its program:

For 80 cents more. The Economist, 15 August 2002: a journalist's account of TEHIP's effect in Tanzania. **http://www.economist.com/World/Africa/ displaystory.cfm?story_id=1280587**

The Publisher

The International Development Research Centre is a public corporation created by the Parliament of Canada in 1970 to help researchers and communities in the developing world find solutions to their social, economic, and environmental problems. Support is directed toward developing an indigenous research capacity to sustain policies and technologies developing countries need to build healthier, more equitable, and more prosperous societies.

IDRC Books publishes research results and scholarly studies on global and regional issues related to sustainable and equitable development. As a specialist in development literature, IDRC Books contributes to the body of knowledge on these issues to further the cause of global understanding and equity. The full catalogue is available at **http://www.idrc.ca/books**.